The Pathway to a Diet-Free Life

SASHA CRAIG-TAYLOR

VTCT, C&G, ITEC

ISBN-13: 978-1482064087

CONTENTS

INTRODUCTION - THE NINE BASIC NEEDS

There is much publicity at present, about the rising epidemics of obesity-related diabetes, heart disease and cancer and one of the biggest culprits is our diet. The food industry makes a vast profit, processing cheap, tasty food, frequently out of cheap, dubious ingredients.

We lead busy lives and it is very convenient to buy ready-made meals, keep them in our freezers and heat them in our microwaves. Why would we want to spend an hour cooking a meal with fresh ingredients when we can have a hot meal on the table within a few minutes of getting home from work? We can experience cuisine from all over the world, from exotic curries to tasty Chinese dishes, all at the click of a switch.

Convenience foods are just that – convenient. If we are hungry we can just pop a few biscuits in our mouths, eat a muffin or two or chew on a snack bar. If you have a good look around your local supermarket, you will realise that the majority of its food products are convenience foods. Take away the fresh meat and fish, milk, butter and cheese, and the fresh fruit and vegetables and the rest are convenience foods. Note, I didn't say 'junk' because most of it is nutritious, but the problem is that it is refined and laced with food additives, which stop it decaying, separating out or changing colour. Food additives also disguise the taste of heavily processed ingredients.

My definition of junk food it ‘food which has very little nutritional value, is potentially harmful, is addictive and can make you ill. Included in this section are sweets, fizzy drinks, cakes and biscuits, crisps and savoury snacks and anything else that is high fat, high sugar, high salt and low fibre. Most people, when asked love to eat some or all of these junk foods, particularly the younger generation, some of whom practically live on them.

I was reminiscing recently, about the birth of my first child and all the different feelings that went through my mind when she arrived in the world. For nine months I had watched and felt her grow, knowing that she was safe and warm inside my growing tummy. As she grew I would stroke her through my skin and sing to her. Even before she was born I had a very special kind of love for her.

Finally, she emerged, after a fourteen hour labour, and as soon as her head appeared I became anxious for her safety. Could she breathe ... was the cord wrapped around her neck ... would she be distressed? Thankfully, all was well and she thrived, but I’ll never forget the feeling that this perfect little being was now in the big wide world, helpless and defenceless.

Human babies are born so helpless because they are not well developed – unlike a foal, or lamb, for example, which can get up and walk almost immediately. If a baby stayed in the uterus until it could fend for itself it would be far too big to be born.

Newborns can do very little. They can grip and suckle and if they are uncomfortable they soon let you know. A baby’s cry cannot be ignored.

We all have nine basic needs:

1. To breathe (respiration)
2. To eat (nutrition)
3. To drink (hydration)
4. To maintain temperature and organ function (homeostasis)
5. To sleep (somnolence)
6. To experience physical affection (touch)
7. To be mentally and physically stimulated (stimulation)
8. To keep clean (cleansing)
9. To fight pests and diseases (immunity)

As soon as a baby emerges he is encouraged to breathe, his face and mouth are cleaned, and he is wrapped up to keep him warm and make him feel secure. His mother's first instinct is to hold him close to her and maybe to feed him.

I used to instinctively talk to my new baby, even though she couldn't understand and it wasn't long before she fixed her gaze on me. The last two of her basic needs became apparent very quickly – the first dirty nappy, with the need to clean her skin, and a few weeks later, a yeast infection, which made her sore and needed an antifungal cream. If I had not been driven to deal with all her basic needs, she would not have survived.

And so began my daughter's journey in the world. I did my best to look after her, to keep her safe and nourished, but she, like most children, had the usual falls, cuts, bruises, infections and times of unhappiness and emotional turmoil. It doesn't matter how hard you try, you can't protect your children all the time.

Going back to my early memories, I was puzzling over why we are so caring about newborn babies and yet we don't look after ourselves. How often do we skip a meal because we are trying to lose weight, forget to drink, breathe smoke filled air, burn our skins in the sun, eat and drink chemical additives, get too hot or too cold or ignore and infection until it has taken hold?

I would be the first one to admit doing all of these things. Some needs, like lack of human contact were out of my control – the same goes for air pollution – both my parents smoked in the house. Having only limited kisses and cuddles as a baby, I was not a happy child and as I grew older, people picked up on my body language, which led to bullying, both by children and adults.

Thankfully now I am an adult I am able to understand, and cope with, the ways of other people and my self-esteem has grown. But there were many years when I did not care about myself or my body – the temple of my soul.

Following the death of my partner, some fourteen years ago, I started to neglect my diet and lived on junk food. It wasn't long before I started to feel unwell. My skin itched, I lost weight, I had a foggy brain, I was depressed and I had frequent infections. I lived like this for several years until I was lucky enough to find love again. It was then that I started my voyage of research and discovery.

I read everything I could get my hands on, wanting to know what I had been doing wrong to make myself feel ill, and was shocked at what I learnt. The day I read my first health book was the first step on my pathway to good health.

I have divided this book into nine sections – one for each basic need. Some things I have written you may already know, but just need reminding – some things will be disturbing. I hope however that you will get the incentive you need to change your life for the better.

Once you are eating good food, eliminating additives from your diet, changing your environment and exercising you will realise what you have been missing. Of course, if you are feeling unwell and have not yet had a check-up with your doctor, I advise you to do so, before you make any changes.

I would like to take you along the pathway to a healthier life. Even if you are happy about your weight I hope to inspire you to make the changes necessary to:

a. keep your body a healthy weight
b. make you feel good, both physically and emotionally.

You may be obese – you may be anorexic – in both cases eating has taken control of your life, and you are missing out on so many opportunities to relax and enjoy life.

I speak from experience as I have been through periods of anorexia in the past. I know the feelings of guilt and the longing to control my body, the feeling that I didn't deserve nice food, the worry that if I ate too much one day I would have to starve the next day.

Obesity also brings similar feelings – guilt, frustration, depression, low self-esteem and the constant desire to give up and put up with your weight problem.

There are hundreds, if not thousands, of diet books and diet plans on the market, most of which will work for a while but which eventually fail. The only way to attain your correct weight is to eat good fresh food and continue to do so - for the rest of your life.

As already stated, we need to meet our eight basic needs in order to thrive. On our pathway to a healthier life I will tackle each of these needs and help you to understand what you might need to do to improve your chances of a healthier life.

1. RESPIRATION

Deep breathing eases depression and lethargy

The first necessity for a newborn baby is to breathe – good clean air. You wouldn't dream of blowing cigarette smoke into a baby's face, would you? We know polluted air is dangerous to health and yet when we are adults we deliberately smoke.

Breathing is the most vital need for all oxygen dependent creatures. Oxygen dissolved in the blood reacts with blood glucose to produce energy. The brain and heart cannot function if they are deprived of oxygenated blood for more than 6 to 8 minutes and we only maintain full oxygen saturation in our blood for about a minute, if breathing stops.

Recently I asked a group of people to imagine where they would like to be, if they could go anywhere on the planet, to relax. Sixty two percent said they would go to a tropical beach, eighteen percent said they would go for a walk in the countryside, twelve percent said they would walk through a forest, five percent said they would lie in the garden, one said he would go round an art gallery and two said they would soak in the bath.

Not one said they would have a bonfire, go for a smoke, have a barbeque or go anywhere where the air was polluted. Our ancient ancestors, the apes, lived in the forests, where trees and shrubs cleansed and purified the air. Our hunter-gatherer cousins also lived in fresh air. We instinctively crave fresh air. We use perfumes to disguise the smells that permeate all around us in our modern polluted environment. Our instinct tells us that if something smells bad, it is unhealthy for us.

So, as we start our journey along the pathway to a healthier and diet-free life I would like you to imagine that you are entering a vast forest, following the trail that many animals have made. Smell the air, feel its freshness wafting all around you, listen to the birds and feel the calmness and energy from the trees. Stand still and take a deep breath.

Here are a couple of suggestions for improving your lung capacity, oxygen saturation and health. A well oxygenated body digests food better and could help you to maintain a healthy weight. Conversely, shallow breathing, poor posture and constant stress leads to retention of toxins and body fat.

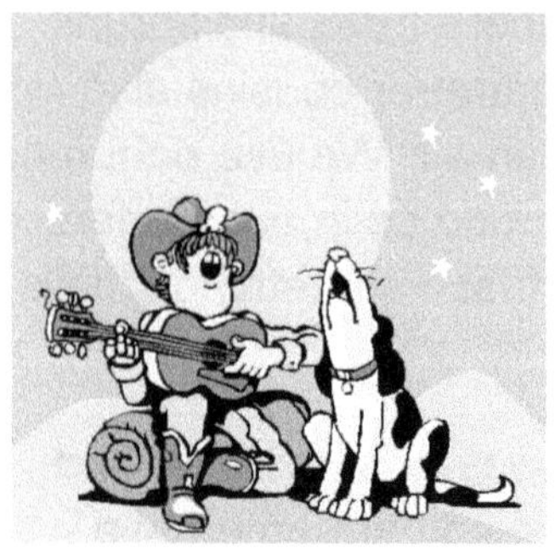

1(a). BREATHE DEEPLY AND SING

Singing and making music are unique to the human race. Birds sing, but not usually for pleasure, they are defending their territory or seeking a mate. Apes don't sing – if they fancy a lady they flex their muscles, beat up the competition and take liberties whenever they can.

Humans are more sophisticated than that. Because of our social customs and taboos we have to be a lot more subtle than apes, and singing shows how fit and clever we are – so does dancing. The better we can sing and dance, the more we impress people, because most of us have music in our souls – beautiful music is a thing of pleasure. Incidentally, music affects our heart rate as well and many pop songs have a beat around 70 to 80 beats a minute – the speed of our hearts when we are stimulated.

There are increasing research results to show that singing is good for your health. It exercises major muscle groups in the upper body. It improves your cardiovascular system and oxygenates your body, making you feel more alert.

Singing is an aerobic activity which reduces stress, increases longevity and improves overall health. Deep breathing increases the airflow in the upper respiratory tract, reducing the risk of bacterial infection, colds and flu. It also improves motor control and coordination, and neurological functioning.

Above all, singing improves the way people feel about themselves – it increases feelings of wellbeing and can help you to overcome pain. Singing in a choir helps people to socialize and it is proven that the sound vibrations of music can calm and relax the brain – hence the recent trend of playing classical music school children.

Deep breathing improves our blood circulation. There is a network of vessels, as vast as our circulatory system, which runs close to our blood vessels and carries lymphatic fluid around our bodies. Lymph is a colorless fluid containing white blood cells, which bathes the tissues and drains through the lymphatic system into the bloodstream. It protects and cleanses our bodies by engulfing invaders and taking them to cleaning stations called lymph nodes, which are situated all around our bodies. When lymph is not flowing effectively you can experience aches and pains because carbon dioxide and waste products build up in your body's tissues and irritate the nerves.

It is a well-known fact that Yogic deep-breathing techniques are very effective in handling depression. When you breathe, the expansion of your rib cage has a pumping action on your lymphatic system. When you are stressed, the tightening of the muscles in your neck and shoulders hinders this process.

Deep breathing helps to clear the lungs of carbon dioxide and fill all the tiny air sacs with life-giving oxygen. It stretches the lungs and improves our brain function, our eyes and the rest of our bodily functions.

What better way to breathe deeply than to sing? It doesn't matter if you sing out of tune, it is the process of holding your breath and letting it out as a song, that does us good. It makes us feel good (even if it irritates your neighbours) and helps us to think clearly.

If you really don't want to sing try this exercise:

Breathe in for one second, hold your breath for one second, and breathe out slowly for one second. Then do the same thing with two seconds, then three, increasing the periods of time between breathing in, holding and breathing out.

I do this form of Yogic breathing whenever I feel stressed or can't get to sleep. I can comfortably hold my breath for ten seconds, getting my breathing rate down to twice a minute. Another form of Yogic breathing is closing one nostril while you breathe in through the other. Reverse this for breathing out. Do ten inhalations on one side and ten on the other side. This is thought to stimulate both hemispheres of your brain.

If you enjoy underwater swimming you are probably a seasoned deep breather. Asthma sufferers have been found to greatly benefit from swimming, as holding the breath fills the lungs and opens up the airways.

If you really value your lungs and the purity of the air you breathe change your spray deodorant for a roll on, and in any case switch to a natural one, as chemicals seep into the lymph nodes under the arms and have been linked to breast cancer. It is difficult not to breathe in the spray from aerosol deodorants, anyway, and you don't really want extra chemicals in your lungs.

The same goes for plug-in air fresheners, they emit chemicals into the air all the time and affect your air quality.

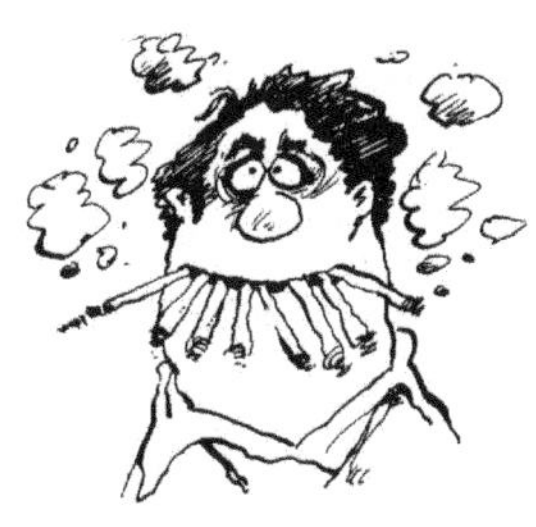

1(b). GIVE UP SMOKING

> *Carbon monoxide—the colorless, odourless, deadly gas present in automobile exhaust—is present in cigarette smoke in more than 600 times the concentration considered safe in industrial plants.*

I firmly believe that plants are not only very sensitive to their surroundings but can also respond to humans as well. I read an amazing book, years ago, called 'The secret Life of Plants' (Tompkins and Bird). They described how plants can respond to human emotions and how their signals can be monitored. If, on your journey along the pathway, you want to smoke a cigarette, think how the surrounding plants might feel about the sudden pollution of their air.

If you are a smoker you don't need reminding of the unbelievable risks of smoking. Some people live to a ripe old age, having smoked most of their lives – they seem to have a genetic resistance to the harm caused by smoking. But 90% of people over 45 say that they would never have started to smoke if they had their time again. It increases the risks of heart disease, stroke, lung cancer and chronic bronchitis. About half of all smokers die early from smoking-related diseases.

There are over 4,000 chemicals in cigarettes - 51 of them are known to be carcinogenic, or cancer causing. In all kinds of cancer, abnormal, mutated body cells keep dividing, forming cancerous tumours or blood chemistry. The carbon monoxide in cigarette smoke robs your body of oxygen and the chemicals inhibit the absorption of nutrients from your food.

If, by writing these things down, just one smoker amongst my readers decides to quit, then it has all been worthwhile. Nicotine is incredibly addictive – one of the most addictive substances known to man. It is no wonder that people find it so difficult to give up. There are many treatments on offer – hypnotherapy, acupuncture, nicotine patches, substitute cigarettes, medication, counselling, aversion therapy and 'cold turkey' where you just decide on a set day that enough is enough. Putting your cigarette money in a piggy bank will soon make you realise how much you were spending on cigarettes.

My parents both smoked and as a child I had many throat and ear infections. I knew smoking was bad – I hated the fuggy atmosphere in the house, the yellowing paintwork and awful smell.

My mother would get me to walk to the village shop, often in the dark, to fetch her cigarettes – how I hated it, especially as I was afraid of the dark!

When I was an adult, however, I got my own back – I caught Asian flu and unintentionally gave it to my mother. She nearly died, as her lungs were full of tar and she was unfit. She lay in bed for weeks and weeks – at times she seemed to be delirious. My father insisted on nursing her himself so she received no medical help and no antibiotics.

Thankfully she recovered – she is now 92 years old, and apart from weak lungs and asthma she is still fine. The only good thing about this story is that after six weeks of being unable to smoke she kicked the habit and never smoked again. In fact, she is the first to complain if there is a smoker nearby.

If you want to give up smoking try getting professional help. The UK Government is at last being proactive in helping people to quit. Smoking puts a huge strain on the National Health system and I'm sure it costs more to treat smokers than the tax that is levied from the sale of cigarettes.

Another thing to bear in mind is the pollution to the atmosphere around you, when you smoke. Passive smoking is almost as harmful as actually smoking a cigarette. If you don't care about your own health, please consider the health of those around you, particularly children.

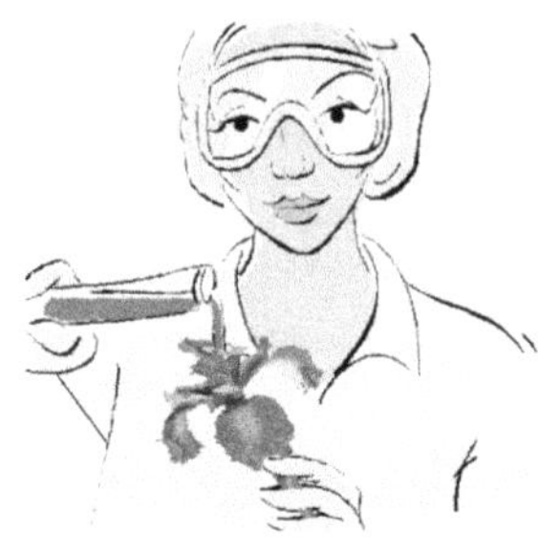

1(c). AVOID CHEMICAL AIR FRESHENERS

Air fresheners contain a multitude of toxic chemicals

Most people live in various forms of housing these days. Whether we live in a mansion, or one small, poorly furnished room we are sheltered from the weather – rain, wind, snow ... and anything else that the climate throws at us. Because of this, the air quality is not as good as living in the open air. And like it or not, we share our living space with a whole host of bacteria, viruses, yeasts, moulds and creepy crawlies.

Winter is the time when all these organisms are normally killed off or sent into dormancy by the cold (if you live in a cold climate) but because we live in heated, enclosed spaces they thrive and live alongside us. Far from shutting down for the winter they thrive because most of our homes are not only warm but moist as well. Breathing and perspiring, alone, moistens the air, as does using the kettle, washing and drying our clothes, having baths and showers and using sinks and toilets.

Our beds, soft furnishings and carpets are an ideal habitat for dust mites and moths (scavengers) lice and bed bugs (blood suckers). Dust mites lurk mainly in our mattresses and pillows, feeding on our dead skin, which we shed constantly. We have roughly 1.6 billion skin cells and between 30,000 and 40,000 of them fall off every hour. Over a twenty-four hour period, we lose almost a million skin cells. In one year, you'll shed more than 8 pounds (3.6 kilograms) of dead skin.

We're all familiar with the dust that settles on everything. Some people dust their furniture every day – some wait until they can write their names in it! Did you know that most of that dust is made from skin cells? Some of it is also the remains of dead creepy crawlies and their faeces. Dust doesn't just settle on shiny surfaces, it coats everything, including our carpets, curtains and flooring. It is this delicious dust that feeds the dust mites and it is their faeces that can cause allergies, such as runny nose and asthma.

Living, as we do, in enclosed spaces, unless we keep our windows open all the time our homes develop a smell. We all have a natural smell anyway, just like the rest of the animal kingdom – tracker dogs demonstrate that clearly. Our smell is governed by the presence of oil in our skin, what we eat, what cleaning and personal hygiene products we use, and our natural hormones.

This also applies to our furnishings and clothing. Our homes are often filled with cooking smells, which linger in the air and fabrics. Cleaning products are usually highly perfumed and these cocktails of different perfumes also add to our homes' smell.

To tackle these smells about 75% of people use air fresheners. In the USA air fresheners make more than one billion dollars in profits. They come in many forms, from solid gel, aerosols, powder filled sachets, perfumed drawer liners and plug-ins.

As a therapist I use a variety of scents to help my clients and they are all from natural plant sources. Natural plant aromas have been proven to affect our mood and many have healing properties. Lavender, in particular, is relaxing and antiseptic. If you are stressed and can't sleep, a little pure lavender oil can really help.

Plants produce these natural oils to defend themselves from pests and diseases and we can use them to help us too. Unfortunately some of these oils are very expensive to extract so most air fresheners are made from artificial chemicals and pollutants, which can threaten our health. A recent study concluded that many air fresheners contain chemicals that could cause developmental and reproductive problems, especially for young children. Some contain phthalates - chemicals that act as plastic softeners to hold fragrances.

Other chemicals present are formaldehyde, petrochemicals, p-dichlorobenzene, ethylene-based glycol ethers, and terpenes (derived from citrus oils that are not inherently dangerous, but react with ozone to form formaldehyde). These pollutants are often released more or less continuously.

If you use mothballs, their main ingredient is 1,4 dichlorobenzene and it is also is present in many air fresheners. This chemical can reduce lung capacity and may hasten respiratory diseases.

I became aware of the problems of air fresheners a few years ago, when I developed asthma, headaches, a blocked nose and brain fog. I used to keep a plug-in air freshener close to the bedroom and couldn't understand why I was feeling so poorly.

In the summer time, when the windows were kept open I felt better, so I quickly realised that air pollutants were to blame. After further research I binned all the chemical air fresheners. Now I have an electric fan air freshener into which I put a few drops of my favourite essential oils – lavender, tangerine, eucalyptus or cedar wood. As essential oils are antiseptic my air freshener also helps to reduce bacteria.

I also have an air purifier in the bedroom. This low powered unit has a heated ceramic plate inside and it destroys harmful organisms. My asthma and allergies are now much improved.

If you have any black mould in your home you need to cure the damp problem and kill the mould, because its spores are harmful and can cause health problems in children. It has a characteristic smell, too, which is unpleasant.

To minimise odours I recommend using proper ventilation, pots of baking soda, and leaving coffee grounds or lemon peels in troublesome areas. Baking soda is particularly effective in fridges. Just pour some into a small open container and leave it in there to absorb the smells. You can change it every two to three months to keep it working effectively.

Incidentally, I use baking soda as an effective deodorant. I was concerned about the potentially harmful chemicals in deodorants and their link to breast cancer so I now mix my own deodorant. I just use E45 cream to which I add a little baking soda. It's a little gritty to use but it does the job perfectly – and is very cheap! Baking soda is also an effective household cleaner.

2. NUTRITION

Starving your body causes weight gain

I have listed twenty suggestions and guidelines to help you to positively change your health and in particular your weight (whether you are overweight or underweight).

By following a healthy diet and eliminating toxins, damaged trans-fats and excess sugar from your diet, your body should soon start to function normally, shedding unwanted fat and giving you more energy.

Going back to our walk along the pathway through the forest, if after a while you feel hungry, which would you rather eat – a mixture of chemicals, heat damaged food and gloopy fat, or freshly picked fruit from the trees?

Be patient with yourself as you change to a healthier diet – fat laid down by bad diet can be hard to shift and you need to be focused. Don't give up - at the end of your journey you will feel better, have a longer life expectancy and have more confidence.

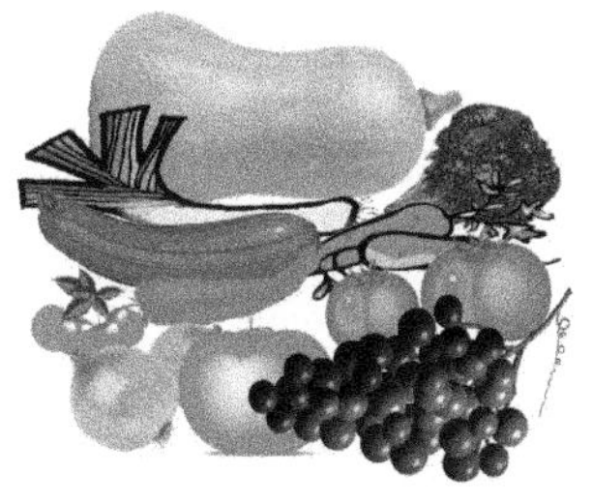

2(a). EAT NOURISHING FOOD AND EAT WHEN YOU ARE HUNGRY

Did you ever see a fat wild chimpanzee? True, some apes have large abdomens, especially gorillas, but that is because they need a vast amount of digestive tract to break down the cellulose in their vegetarian diet. But if you look at their arms and legs, they are muscular but not full of stored fat.

Millions of years ago our distant ancestors were great apes, who foraged in the forests. As we evolved we moved onto the plains of Africa. Humans and apes are all classified as hominidae, and our four distant cousins are chimpanzees, bonobos, gorillas and orangutangs.

We humans come in a huge variety of sizes, shapes and skin colour. Even our hair type and skull shapes are different, according to where in the world our ancestors came from. We seem to have inherited an assortment of residual characteristics from our ape ancestors too. Some African men have very dark skin, small ears and thick necks, like gorillas. Some people have red hair, like orangutangs. Some have large ears, which get longer as they age, like chimps, and some are less hairy, longer legged, and lighter skinned, like bonobos (who, incidentally, are sex mad, like humans!)

Some races of people have flat faces, others have heavy jaws or high cheekbones. The human race has changed according to where they migrated in the world. The fact they we walk upright on two legs has affected our distribution of hair and the shapes of our faces. Dark skin protects us from the sun's ultraviolet rays, oriental eye shape protects our eyes, again from harmful overhead rays. Thick woolly hair protects our heads from sunburn and rain, and light skin enables us to use sunlight to make vitamin D for strong bones. A large brow rim with bushy eyebrows, also protects our eyes from sweat and strong light, as we look ahead, to spot possible prey in the distance.

The main difference between apes and men is our intelligence, and our ability to remember the past, think about the present and plan for the future. Hence, by anticipating the future, we are food hoarders. Chimps, and the rest of the animal kingdom, are as intelligent as they need to be. Apes have an amazing recall off exactly where all the best food is and remember their environment without the need of a sat nav.

When a chimp gets out of bed in the morning, it doesn't go to the fridge or cupboard to get out a pack of cereal and a bottle of milk. Although many members of the animal kingdom do store food, apes do not as they live in a plentiful environment. There are roots, nuts, shoots, leaves and fruit, often in close proximity. All they have to do is get out of bed and go and find food.

Life for them, however, isn't that easy. Chimps are very choosy about what they eat and they can't just reach out and pick the leaves from their dormitory tree. They have a mind map of all the fruiting trees in the forest and they often have to do a fair bit of walking, clambering and climbing to find what they fancy. When they do find a tree full of ripe fruit they will eat as much as they can, taking advantage of the abundancy of food. They will then rest, leave the food to digest and not eat again until they are hungry again.

What has all this to do with 'eating when you're hungry?' We are told to start the day with breakfast, first thing in the morning, whether we are hungry or not, because our metabolism is at its most efficient then. If you were a chimp you would have to do some foraging before you could eat. I came to the conclusion some time ago that the best time to eat breakfast is when you feel hungry – not ravenous, but when you are really thinking about food. This may be as soon as you get up, but if not, by all means have a drink and then eat when you do feel hungry.

This could be awkward if you are working. You can't exactly get out a bowl of porridge in the middle of a board meeting. This is where planning comes in. If you look at the ingredients on a breakfast bar wrapper it will probably contains a lot of sugar, refined carbohydrates and other chemical additives – even if it states it is 'healthy'.

The best natural convenience foods are in the fruit and nut group. It is easy to take a container of natural nibbles with you to eat. This could contain a small handful of natural (not roasted) nuts, and maybe a few raisins, a stick or two of carrot, a banana, strawberries, tangerine segments, apples or pears, to mention a few. These will give you slow release energy for quite a while, but won't over fill your stomach. An alternative is to make your own batch of muesli bars or buy one that is low sugar and additive free.

Every time you feel hungry have a small quantity of healthy food – enough to satisfy your hunger. Once you stop eating processed foods you will get your hunger under control. Just stay away from sweets, crisps, chocolates and fizzy drinks.

There are several types of signal that control your appetite – some tell you when you are hungry and some tell you that your stomach is full. A hormone call Ghrelin is your main hunger signal and other, called Peptide YY, tells you your stomach is full. Of course, if you have eaten a huge meal your stomach will have stretched and you will feel uncomfortably full anyway.

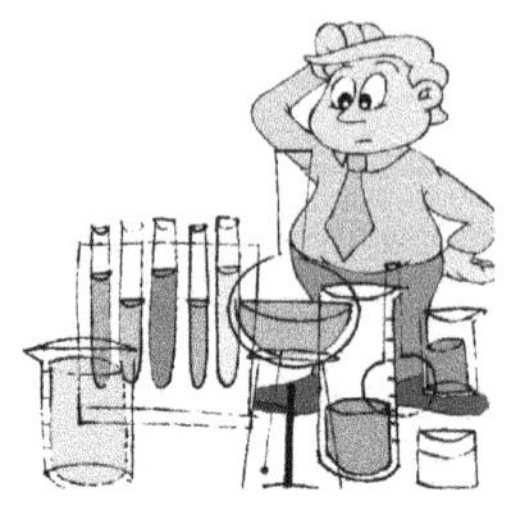

2(b). AVOID ARTIFICIAL SWEETENERS

Artificial sweeteners are made from potentially toxic chemicals

As humans, we crave sweet things. Our brains use a lot of energy and eating sweet food is the quickest way to feed our brains. Many natural foods contain natural sugars. Apart from fruit, these sugars are locked up in long chemical chains and our bodies have to work to extract them and break them down into blood glucose.

Think about sweeteners. Which would you rather eat – some fresh natural fruit or something to which a cocktail of artificial ingredients have been added, including chemical sweetener?

You may think that sugar-free food and drinks are the best alternative to sugar, if you want to lose weight. They may be virtually calorie free but they are not safe to consume for long periods. There is a huge amount of publicity about chemical sweeteners if you want to check this out.

Apart from the sweet poison aspect, the sweetness in artificial sweeteners tricks your brain into thinking you have just taken in sugar and your pancreas releases insulin to deal with it. Some artificial sweeteners, such as aspartamine have been linked with an increased cancer risk, and impaired brain function.

It can get into your brain and joints and make you ill. Aspartame comes in many guises including NutraSweet, Equal, Spoonful, and Equal-Measure. In the USA it has been found to account for 75 percent of adverse reactions to food additives reported to the FDA.

Saccharine is another dubious sweetener. It was first developed in the 1870's and is one of the earliest artificial sweeteners. It is made from derivatives of coal tar. Its main ingredients are anthranilic acid (used as a corrosive agent for metal), nitrous acid, sulphur dioxide, chlorine, and ammonia.

There is one natural sweetener, called Stevia, a member of the sunflower family, and it is made from the plant's leaves. It is very sweet, is completely calorie free, but does leave a lingering after-taste. It appears to be the safest of the sweeteners.

For a sweet taste, use sugar and honey (in moderation)

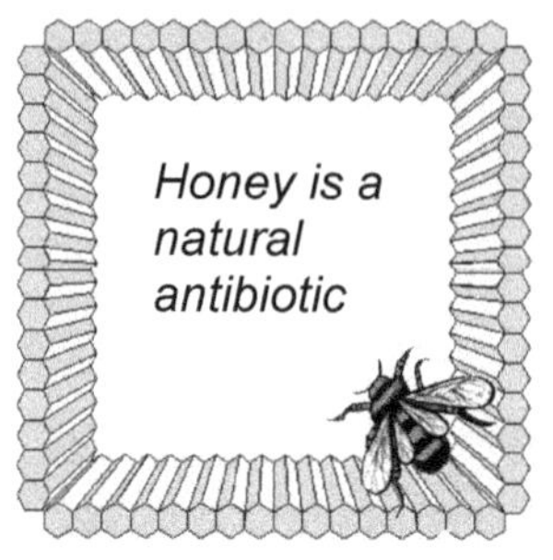

2(c). EAT HONEY

Honey is the most natural sweetener you can eat and has been known to humans for thousands of years. Although slightly more calorific than sugar (a teaspoon of honey has 22 calories, and a teaspoon of sugar has 16) you need less of it, as it is sweeter. Honey is antiseptic and cleansing. It has to be, to protect the tightly packed bees in their nests, from bacterial and viral infections. Manuka honey is well known for it's wound healing properties and is used to treat skin ulcers. Honey and salt are often used to treat skin infections that don't respond to infections. Incidentally, maggots are also used to clean up dead and infected tissue.

Honey helps to treat digestive problems such as diarrhoea, indigestion, stomach ulcers and gastroenteritis. Because it contains a cocktail of valuable enzymes, proteins, vitamins and minerals, it breaks down slower than sugar and therefore does not cause the pancreas to release insulin as quickly as sugar.

Sugar is often classified as having empty calories, whereas honey contains substances that can aid in digestion. It also contains anti-oxidants, which can protect your body from free radicals – particles which damage your cells.

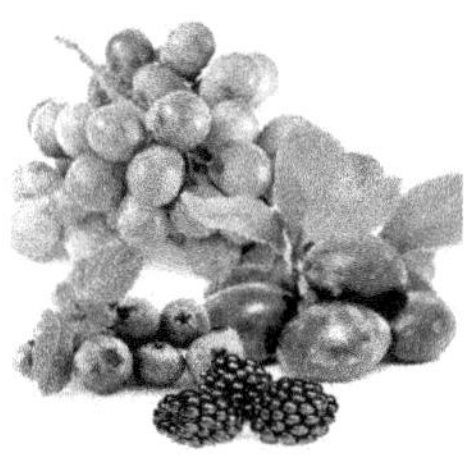

2(d). EAT FOOD WHICH IS RICH IN ANTIOXIDANTS

Oxidation occurs when oxygen reacts with something and causes it to degenerate. A good example would be when the oxygen in air reacts with iron to form rust. Oxygen is vital for or body's cells. Put very simply, it combines with the food we have eaten to produce heat. The bi-products of this process are carbon dioxide and water, which we eliminate from our bodies. However, up to 2% of oxygen molecules in our blood stream lose one of their electrons and become unstable. They try to grab missing electrons from our cells, setting up a chain reaction. These unstable atoms are called free radicals and they damage our cells.

> *Antioxidants protect our bodies from rogue oxygen atoms*

Our immune systems are very good at mopping up and disposing of damaged cells (as well as dead bacteria and other detritus) but as we get older they become less efficient. Every day millions of our body cells die and not all of these are replaced. It is this diminishing of replacement cells that causes slow degeneration. This is the natural process of ageing. There is much evidence relating cell damage from oxidation and cancer. There is also documentation to show that a healthy, raw-food rich diet, slows down ageing.

Antioxidants are contained in foods which make their own protection against damage from the sun's rays. So nearly all fruits and leaves contain antioxidants. The brighter the colour, the better they are for you.

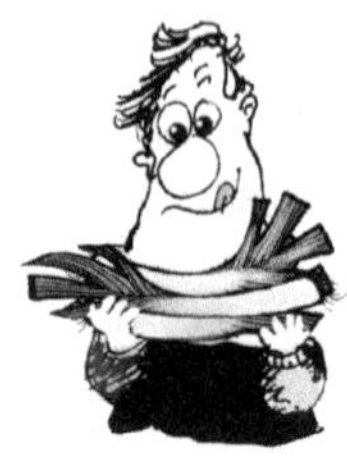

2(e). EAT AS MUCH RAW FOOD AS POSSIBLE

Did you ever see any member of the animal kingdom lighting a fire, filling a pan full of meat and vegetables, lacing it with salt and other flavourings and cooking it? It's a silly question, I know, but that is what humans do. Everything living on the planet survives by eating some other living thing – raw!

Imagine, if you were visiting a local restaurant to have a relaxing meal with a friend. There are two food counters – one is nicely laid out with a variety of fresh salads, potatoes, tomatoes, cold meats, etc. and the other has a variety of chemicals and food that had been cooked until it had lost all its colour and flavour. Which would you choose? Would you fill your plate with the natural food or would you experiment with the chemicals until the processed food looked and smelt good?

In a way, that is what food manufacturers do for us. They cook food so that it will keep for long periods and it is safe to package, but then they have to add chemicals to stop it from deteriorating or tasting bad.

> *We have about twenty one feet of small intestines – for digesting fibre*

Heating food damages or destroys its vitamins and minerals and breaks down its fibre. In addition, if you eat a food that has been *heated* beyond a certain temperature (unique to each food) or if a food is *processed* (refined, chemicals added, etc.) this always causes a rise in the number of white cells in the blood. The white cells are part of your immune system and increase when the body is threatened by 'foreign bodies'.

Cooking food, however, has many advantages for us – it kills harmful bacteria, softens food, enables us to store it, makes it easier (and faster) to eat and digest, and makes it taste good. But it also damages food. When you eat cooked food it is dead. Its life-force has gone, along with much of its goodness.

The life-force angle is an interesting one. Every living thing has an electromagnetic force in and around it. This electromagnetism controls the exchange of gases and nutrients, cell repair and regeneration, heart beat, brain activity – to name but a few. It can be seen in Kirlian photography – a photographic technique that shows the electromagnetic forces around a living thing. Why not *add* to your natural energy by taking in the plant energy in raw food?

And why not eat a good helping of the myriads of essential vitamins and minerals contained in plants? Some trace elements, such as magnesium, calcium, potassium, iron, zinc, copper, manganese, iodine, chromium, selenium and molybdenum are essential for a healthy body.

Abnormally low levels of these trace elements in your body could cause the following disorders:

magnesium/potassium - heart disease
selenium - cancer and heart disease
iodine – hypothyroidism (low thyroid)
iron - anaemia
chromium - diabetes
manganese - epilepsy
zinc - immunity problems, infertility, behaviour problems, etc.

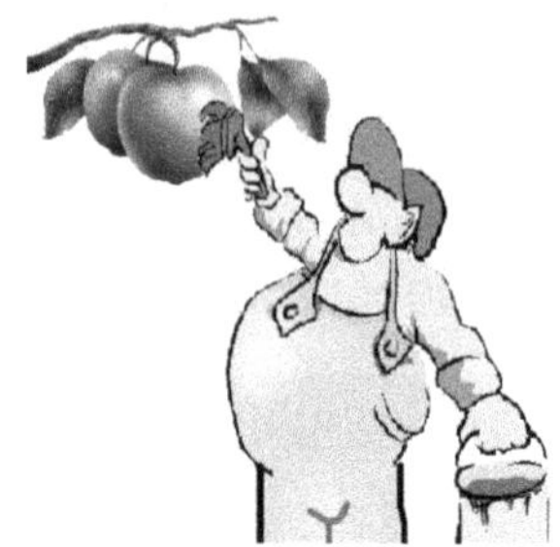

2(f). EAT NATURALLY COLOURED FOOD

Think about the meal you last ate. Was it beige? Was it lacking in colour? Let's think of a beige meal – breakfast cereal and milk, macaroni cheese, maybe, with rice pudding. Or a cheese sandwich on white bread, or sausage and mashed potato. True, there are some vitamins, carbohydrates and proteins in the meal but they are just about as far from natural as they can be.

Our ape cousins live on raw fruit and vegetables (and chimps eat raw meat and eggs as well) and that is what our digestive systems were designed to handle

The colour in fruit skins protects it from ultraviolet radiation

Follow the food rainbow – and I don't mean go for artificial colours – pick your weekly menu from all the colours of the rainbow – red tomatoes, orange butternut squash, creamy bananas, fresh green spinach, blueberries, purple plums – there is a huge variety of foods to choose from.

If you're not used to eating natural foods you may find your digestive system becomes overactive at first, but keep trying raw food and your body will soon adjust.

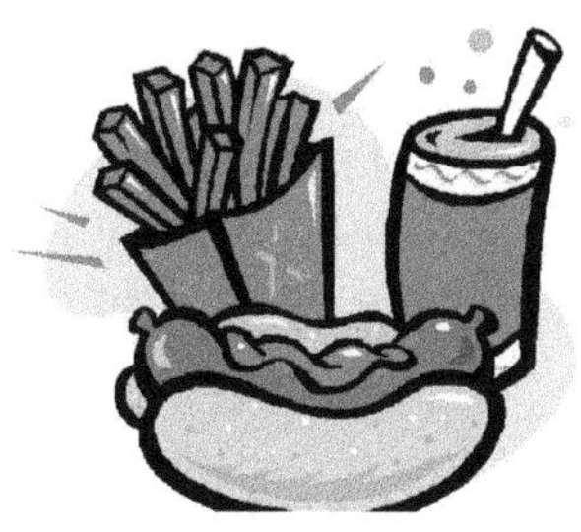

2(g). STOP EATING READY-MADE MEALS AND JUNK FOOD

Eating junk food is addictive and makes you gain weight

The more processes food has been through, the less beneficial it is. In fact there is plenty of evidence to show that it is positively harmful. There is an epidemic of obesity in the US, Canada, the UK and Europe. About 75% of Americans and Canadians are overweight or obese and one quarter of UK adults are clinically obese. The rest of the so-called civilized world are following the trend – the more fast food outlets being opened in developing countries the higher the rise in obesity.

The main culprit is undoubtedly processed food. It contains saturated fats, salt, sugar, chemicals, refined carbohydrates and is addictive. The reason processed food is addictive is because it usually contains milk and wheat flour. Everyone knows that cigarettes and alcohol are addictive but did you know that some food is addictive too?

Some prepared foods contain physically addictive substances such as beta-carbolines and mutagenic heterocyclic amines. But many of them also contain milk and wheat flour. The reason that food manufacturers add these everyday ingredients to food is because they know that they contain opioid peptides, which can be addictive.

Opioid peptides are amino acids that mimic the effect of opiates in the brain. An opiate is a chemical substance that acts as a sedative. Opioid peptides are also produced by the body itself, like endorphins – the chemicals released when you exercise, have sex or meditate.

Endorphins relieve stress and reduce pain. Natural brain opioid peptides play an important role in motivation, emotion, attachment behaviour, the response to stress and pain, and the control of food intake.

When you are addicted to these amino acids and you stop eating the food that contains them, your levels drop and you can become emotional and stressed. Your body screams at you to fix the problem – with more junk food.

Another problem with convenience foods is their added salt. Salt (sodium chloride) is in everything – even breakfast cereals. We need a certain amount of salt each day - an average adult requires an intake of 4.2g salt per day. The minimum requirement is 1.5g. If we eat too much salt we get thirsty. This is because excess sodium in the blood draws water out of our cells and makes us dehydrated. This can be very dangerous, especially if the weather is hot.

A good way to reduce your salt intake is to use 'half salt' which is 50% potassium chloride and 50% sodium chloride. It tastes just the same and the potassium has added health benefits.

Potassium plays an important part in regulation blood acidity, water balance and blood pressure. It is used in the transmission of nerve impulses, the building of muscle tissue and for the beating of your heart. It is also necessary for the metabolism of carbohydrates and proteins.

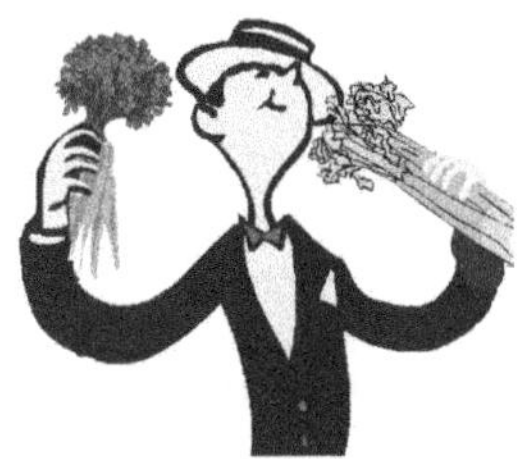

2(h). EAT FIBRE

Eating fibre is essential for a healthy heart

Dietary fibre is vital for a healthy digestive system. Fibre comes from the hard, supportive parts of plants. It is classified as soluble and insoluble – both are important for good health.

Insoluble fibre helps your food to travel through your gut. It gives the food something for your intestinal muscles to push on. Your intestines are surrounded by involuntary muscles, which move in a wavelike motion, pushing food along while digestive enzymes break it down and it is absorbed into your blood stream.

Fibre also helps to sweep the lining of your gut, taking dead cells and bacteria and other detritus for elimination. Without fibre you will get constipated leaving you susceptible to hemorrhoids, hernias and prolapse.

Soluble fibre is fermented in the gut by friendly bacteria and passes through the intestines into the bloodstream. It is thought that it also lowers harmful LDL (low density liproprotein) cholesterol. Fibre is linked to the prevention of heart disease and some cancers, it reduces blood pressure, regulates blood sugar, and aids in weight control.

Food additives cause weight gain and allergies

2(i). AVOID ARTIFICIAL FOOD ADDITIVES

Our bodies are very good at extracting nutrients from whatever we eat but some chemicals in our food are so far removed from anything natural, the body just can't deal with them. Chemical food additives can cause weight gain, joint problems and allergies.

The body has several strategies for dealing with unwanted substances. It's first strategy is to break it down in the liver. Failing that it stores them in body fat, hides them away in your joints, or tries to eliminate them through your skin.

If you had something unpleasant to handle (something rotten or filthy) you would protect your hands by wearing gloves or wrap it in a bag or paper towel before disposing of it. Your body wraps toxic substances in fat and stores it, often round your middle. This is why when you eat a lot of junk food you put on weight and find it very difficult to shed the fat.

Have you ever had achy joints, a persistently runny nose or itchy skin rash? These symptoms point to an allergic reaction. Your body is trying to get an allergen out of your bloodstream through your skin and mucous membranes and your liver is working hard to try to break things down.

When you buy processed food, look at the label. The more unnatural ingredients there are, the less likely it is that the food will be good for your health.

LDL cholesterol can fur up your arteries – HDL can do the reverse

2(j). REDUCE YOUR LDL CHOLESTEROL

Our bodies cannot function without cholesterol, a waxy steroid of fat. It has many functions and is used to make the membrane that covers all our nerves (myelin sheath). Our brains are 60% fat and cholesterol is used to make the cells' membranes.

Cholesterol is a soft, fatty compound belonging to a class of molecules called steroids. It is essential in the formation and maintenance of cell membranes and is mainly produced in the liver, with a small amount coming from the lining of the small intestine. It is used to make bile salts which aid the digestive process and is also transported in the blood plasma. Because it is a fatty substance, the liver binds it to protein ready for transportation in the water based blood, and this is where the word lipoprotein comes from (lipo=fat, + protein).

Cholesterol is classified by its density – high and low. Low density lipoprotein (LDL) is the harmful one. It is small enough to oxidise and build up in your artery linings, thus causing a constriction and clogging up your circulatory system.

High-density lipoproteins are larger in size and they collect and carry cholesterol from the body's tissues to the liver, where it is broken down or recycled. Because HDLs can remove cholesterol from fatty deposits within arteries, and transport it back to the liver for excretion or re-utilisation, they are seen as "good" lipoproteins.

Eating fish can protect you from heart disease and cancer

2(k). EAT MORE ESSENTIAL FATTY ACIDS

There is a theory that at one point in our evolution we took to living in and around the sea. We are very attracted to water, unlike chimps, who can't swim. We also like salty food. Chimps can't hold their breath either. Our body fat is distributed differently too, making it easier for us to float and keep warm in cool water.

Unlike chimps, we rely mostly on fish to get enough omega-3 fatty acid, as we can't synthesis it in our bodies. Most of this fat is found in not only in fish, but also seaweed and algae although it can also be found in some plants and nuts as well

The people of the Mediterranean eat plenty of fish and raw, fresh fruit and vegetables and they are some of the healthiest people in the world. We are guaranteed a calcium-rich diet if we have plenty of fish (especially those with edible bones, like sardines and tinned salmon) and seafood.

Make sure you get your fish from an unpoluted source though, some is harvested from seas that are poluted with heavy metals, such as mercury.

According to the American Heart Association, we should eat fish (particularly oily fish such as mackerel, trout, herring, sardines, tuna, and salmon) at least twice a week.

Omega-3 fatty acids have been shown to reduce inflammation – a condition common in obese people with large amounts of fat around their internal organs.

It may also help to lower the risk of chronic diseases such as heart disease, cancer, and arthritis. Human brains have highly concentrated amounts of omega-3 fatty acids. They are necessary for memory and brain performance and behavioral function. Omega-3 is important for pregnant women to protect their children from vision and nerve problems.

Symptoms of omega-3 fatty acid deficiency include fatigue, poor memory, dry skin, heart problems, mood swings or depression, and poor circulation.

The two other vital omega fatty acids are omega-6 and omega-9. We need to eat these EFA's in the right proportion – taking in twice as much omega-6 as omega-3. Omega-6 can be found in seeds, nuts, grains and seeds, leafy green vegetables and raw pressed vegetable oil.

Omega-9, or monounsaturated oleic and stearic acid, is a non essential fatty acid produced naturally by the body whenever there is enough of either Omega-3 and 6 essential fatty acids.

This fatty acid plays a role in preventing heart disease by lowering cholesterol levels. Other benefits of omega 9 are that it reduces hardening of the arteries and improves immune function.

Most foods contain vitamins and minerals – no food contains them all

2(I). EAT A WIDE VARIETY OF FOODS

Many of us are privileged to be able to buy a huge variety of foods, from fruit and vegetables, nuts and seeds to meat and fish. We have evolved to be omnivorous – like our chimp cousins, but we do have long intestines, indicating that the majority of our diet should be vegetable based.

Herbivores need long intestines in order to break down the cellulose and fibre in their diet. Carnivores have short intestines because meat ferments and putrefies, creating toxins.

There are a few weight loss programs that virtually eliminate carbohydrates from the diet. Carbohydrates break down into sugars to give us energy. If you eat a lot of animal protein instead, your body has to use that instead but the by-products are ketones, which can be very harmful.

It is important that we eat as many different foods as possible in order to get all the nutrients we need. Every food has different nutrients and none of them has all. Vegetables and fruit should form a large part of our diet. In my book 'Why Sugar Makes You Hungry and Dieting Makes You Fat' I talk about the 3-2-1 food plate and I personally believe that our diets should consist of 3 parts fruit and vegetables, 2 parts carbohydrates and 1 part protein (meat or fish) and fats. I have followed this strategy for years and have remained slim and fit.

When you shop for food try to buy fresh as much as possible. The more food additives there are, the less likely it is that it will be good for you. Check the labels on packaged goods. Some of them have a long list of additives, all designed to: make the food palatable, stop it from separating out, keep it from decaying, make it appealing to the eye, and to 'enhance' the taste. Many of these additives are totally unnatural and unlikely to be good for you if you consume them frequently.

If you are vegetarian there are plenty of sources of protein. Although their amino acids are not in the most ideal combination, our bodies can use a variety of them to build our body tissue. Nuts, grains, legumes, tofu and soy, dairy products, eggs, and meat substitutes are ideal meat substitutes.

It is better to eat little and often, with a 3 to 4 hour gap between main meals and snacking on fruit between meals. Fruit is quickly digested and contains fructose, a type of sugar. If you need to lose weight, go for raw carrots or nuts instead.

There is a theory that eating raw fruit at the end of a meal can cause it to ferment, as the digestion of a mixed meal takes far longer, but raw fruit is always better than cooked or canned. Bananas are particularly tasty and easy to eat. They contain potassium 40, which in large doses is radioactive, so don't eat more than a dozen a day! They are also high calorie, although they aid digestion and metabolism.

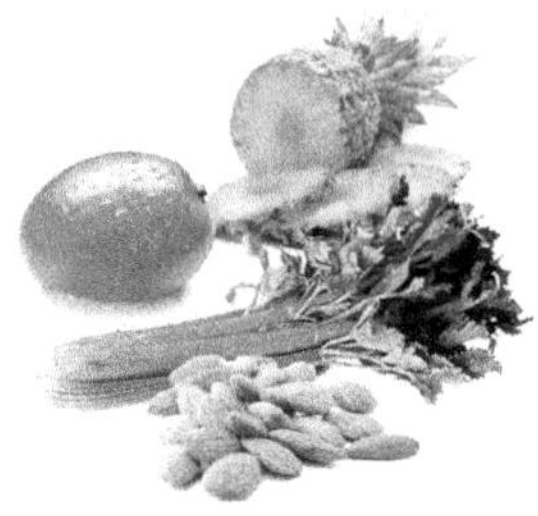

2(m). EAT COMPLEX CARBOHYDRATES

High fibre foods keep you fuller for longer

Carbohydrates are made mainly from carbon and hydrogen and are formed in chains of varying lengths. Carbohydrates are broken down into simple sugars to make blood glucose, which is needed for energy. The longer the chain, the more complex the carbohydrate and the more involved the process it has to go through for the body to use it.

A simple carbohydrate would be sugar, which can even be absorbed through the lining of the mouth. A complex carbohydrate would be wheat, complete with its seed coating and bran.

Complex carbohydrates have plenty of fibre and its takes some time for the body to cut them up into useable short chains. It tends to be bulky, fills the stomach for longer and releases its sugars far more slowly. We have evolved to eat complex carbohydrates.

Simple carbohydrates, like biscuits or cake, are readily available for digestion and conversion into glucose. Because the fibre has been taken away it takes far more of it to fill your stomach, so you eat many more calories before your stomach is full. The sugar is quickly released into the bloodstream and as your blood glucose rises rapidly your pancreas has to release a spike of insulin to deal with it.

The main job of the pancreas is to instruct your cells' membranes to allow the take-up of glucose and storage of any excess. Eating refined food stresses your pancreas, leading to diabetes, as well as making you obese.

The best way to eat carbohydrates is as *unprocessed* as possible – jacket potatoes, raw vegetables, porridge oats, wholemeal bread, and wholegrain pasta and rice – are some examples.

The human brain is 60% fat

2(n). EAT HEALTHY FATS

Our bodies need fats – they are essential for many things, including synthesis of vitamins, keeping us warm, making brain cells and body cells, protecting our nerves, storing energy for lean times, and transporting hormones. Eating fat doesn't necessarily make us fat. It is sugar that is converted into body fat. Fat makes our food palatable and pleasant in texture and life is unpleasant without it.

There is much talk about saturated, unsaturated and polyunsaturated fats. Fats are made from hydrogen, carbon and one oxygen molecule, in chains of various lengths. It is all to do with the shape of the chain and the number of hydrogen atoms that makes a saturated or unsaturated fat – the more hydrogen the more saturated it is.

Trans fats or hydrogenated fats are heat-damaged fats that are used to make up cooking oils and spreads. They are also used in fast food outlets. Vegetable oils are heated to high temperatures and then have hydrogen gas forced through them. This gives the fat a long life so it doesn't go rancid. You can also heat these oils to higher temperatures so they are crisper. Bear in mind, however, that the more food is heated, the more damaged it becomes and the more carcinogenic it becomes.

The result is thick, creamy and gloopy and is widely used over and over again by the fast food industry. Have you ever been past a fast food outlet and smelt the strong smell of the cooking oil? It is quite repulsive. It is often weeks or even months before it is replaced.

Each time hydrogenated oil is heated its atomic structure is damaged more and more. Your body uses this oil to make up your brain and body cells and the result is that many of the cells are unable to function properly. Sticky oil results in sticky cell walls, hindering the transfer of nutrients and gases and inducing the body to make fat cells, storing them around your waist and internal organs. There is a strong link between high consumption of trans-fats and diabetes and cancer.

When you eat oils and fats, use cold pressed virgin oil, such as olive oil, sunflower oil, rice bran oil ... there are many to choose from according to your personal taste. Don't heat it more than once. Eat butter – it tastes better and is more natural. All spreads and oils are calorific so don't eat too much if you want to lose weight, but enjoy what you do eat.

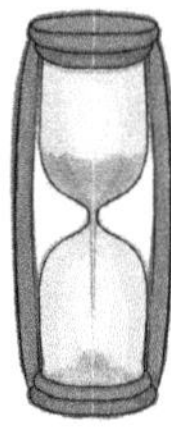

2(o). EAT SLOWLY

Eating releases endorphins – feel good hormones

Our emotional state of mind and the way we digest food are very closely related. If you are tense, your abdominal muscles, both voluntary and involuntary will be tense. This will affect the effectiveness of your digestion. If your digestion is inefficient you will eat more than you need.

Most of us lead busy lives, especially if we are at work. We sit and eat at our desks, looking at our computer screens while we pop a sandwich or snack into our mouths.

A recent study has shown that just by eating slower, people actually take in fewer calories. If you did that, you could lose up to 20 pounds a year without changing your diet. Our brains take about 20 minutes to register when we are full. If we eat fast, we can easily miss the fullness signal. If we eat slowly, we have time to realize we're full, and stop on time.

If you eat slowly, chewing each mouthful thoroughly, you are aiding digestion by mixing amylase in your saliva into the food. This starts to break down carbohydrates even before they reach your stomach. The taste sensations will send pleasure signals to your brain, helping you to relax.

It is far better to eat away from distractions such as computers or TV screens. By eating in a relaxed environment you will become sensitive to your body's signals, your digestion will be more efficient and you will stop eating before you are over-full, helping you to lose excess weight.

When you are eating a meal take smaller mouthfuls, chew slowly and put your knife and fork down in between mouthfuls. Savour each mouthful, tasting the different flavours and feeling the different textures of your food. Sit and talk to your friends and loved ones, by all means but don't discuss stressful subjects.

Eating regularly helps you maintain a healthy weight

2(p). EAT REGULARLY TO MAINTAIN A STABLE BLOOD GLUCOSE LEVEL

Our ancient cousins, the great apes, lived in food abundant conditions and could eat whenever they were hungry. However, during our evolution we moved out of the forests and onto the plains of Africa. This was mainly because the forests diminished, because of the tenacity of the grass. As it spread into the edges of the forests it strangled the sapling trees and gradually worked its way into the undergrowth, making the forests shrink.

Early man was forced to find food elsewhere and hunter-gathering became his new strategy. Food was often not easy to come by and sometimes he would go days before he caught an animal or found a food rich plant. The people without adequate fat storage simply starved and so the fat-storers went on to populate the world. This is now our main problem. Most of us live in abundancy but our fat storage genes are still in operation.

Babies are rarely born fat, and if they are fed breast milk, on demand, they will develop a healthy subcutaneous fat covering, which gets used up when they start crawling and walking. Most children are active and stay a healthy weight. It is only when we start feeding them with refined, calorific food, which is loaded with chemicals, that they become fat – some are dangerously fat at an early age.

What has all this to do with eating regularly, you may ask? It isn't how often we eat but *what* we eat that starts the fat storing problem. And once the problem starts, we try to cope by starving the fat out of our bodies.

Starvation is the trigger for fat storage and we then go into hunter-gatherer mode. Once we have gained a significant amount of internal fat, life will never be the same again. Even if we manage to lose it, our bodies will continue to snatch and grab every spare calorie, in fear of going through lean times, on the plains of Africa.

If you are a parent with young children, this is your opportunity to give them a good chance in life to be a healthy weight in adulthood. The secret for us all is to go back to browser mode and eat good quality, unprocessed food whenever we are hungry.

We enjoy eating a plateful of food, usually about three times a day. This is fine as long as we eat slowly, enjoy good quality food and don't overfill our stomachs. It is far better to eat a smaller meal and have a healthy snack between meals. This keeps your blood glucose steady. If you are ravenous before you eat, your blood glucose will be low and when you do eat, your pancreas will produce too much insulin.

Insulin is the key that instructs your cells to take in glucose. When you have eaten refined food and your stomach is full, your cells will quickly become replete and there will still be plenty of insulin in your bloodstream, with nothing to work on. Your brain senses the high insulin levels and thinks you are hungry. The result is that you keep eating when you don't need to, and thus start storing fat.

It is never too late to change your eating habits. I'm not saying it will be easy, especially if you are carrying a lot of internal fat. Your survival instincts are so strong – your body is protecting you from starving to death. Switching to good quality food is the key to your success. Once you stop feeding your body with refined flour, sugar, trans-fats and chemicals, you will get control of your hunger pangs.

Fresh, high fibre food, which is high in vitamins and minerals will break down slowly in your digestive system and release glucose slowly into your blood making you feel fuller for longer. Your over-worked pancreas will calm down, your over-stretched stomach will shrink to its normal size and you will have more energy.

If you a diabetic, you will need to monitor your blood glucose levels carefully. It may be that your pancreas is completely worn out so you will need to continue with your insulin injections, but the dosage should decrease as you get into a healthy way of eating. In this case it is important to seek medical advice and tell your health practitioner what you are doing.

I have met several people who are no longer diabetic, having switched to a better diet. If you are pre-diabetic, now is the time to change and increase your life expectancy and quality.

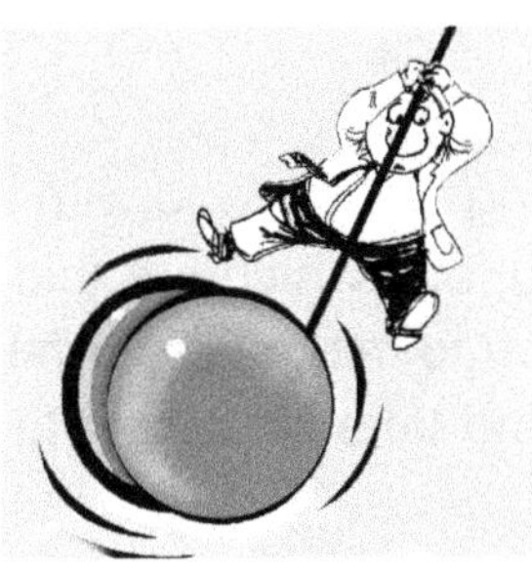

2(q). AVOID YO-YO DIETING

Erratic eating can make you fat

We all do it, don't we – we celebrate a special occasion such as Christmas or a wedding, by eating plenty of rich food and having plenty of alcohol, then we promise ourselves we'll shed the pounds when it's all over.

The peak time for new membership to fitness club and gyms is at the beginning of each year, when people make New Year's resolutions to shed the pounds they have gained over the previous year.

It is a time when we are determined to stick to a diet of celery and lettuce and attend the gym five days a week, but it doesn't last. Our low calorie diet makes us feel depressed and miserable and the gym soon becomes boring. Sure enough, the pounds drop off at first, and we feel pleased with ourselves. We celebrate by having a treat or two and then we gradually return to our original lifestyle. We're busy, we buy ready meals and share lattés and cakes with our friends and for a while we ignore the increasing weight.

As we get older it gets harder and harder to shed excess weight. Years of yo-yo dieting make our bodies lay down internal fat, round our organs – our hearts, livers, stomachs and intestines. From the very first time we go on a low calorie diet our bodies are re-programmed to grab onto extra calories for the rest of our lives. This has even been found to apply to babies in the womb. If their mother diets during pregnancy, she is setting her unborn child up for weight gain when it is older.

There is a problem associated with the eating of junk food with its hydrogenated fats. These fats are damaged fats, which are thick and sticky in texture and our body uses them to make up our fat cells. These cells do not behave normally and take far longer to shed their load.

Another problem with bingeing and starving is that when we binge our fat cells multiply, mainly around our waists. Dieting makes the body give up its fat but now we have far more storage units for the next binge. The next time we put on weight we gain more than the last time, simply because our bodies have more capacity.

If you need to lose weight, do it slowly – a pound or two a week is plenty – and when you reach your ideal weight, eat regularly, with a good quality, high fibre diet.

Factory made bread contains a host of undisclosed additives

2(r). MAKE YOUR OWN BREAD

If you think that a staple food like bread is plain and simple and really good for you, you could be mistaken. The food industry is permitted to use up to sixty chemicals in the making of flour and bread and they don't have to be listed in the ingredients.

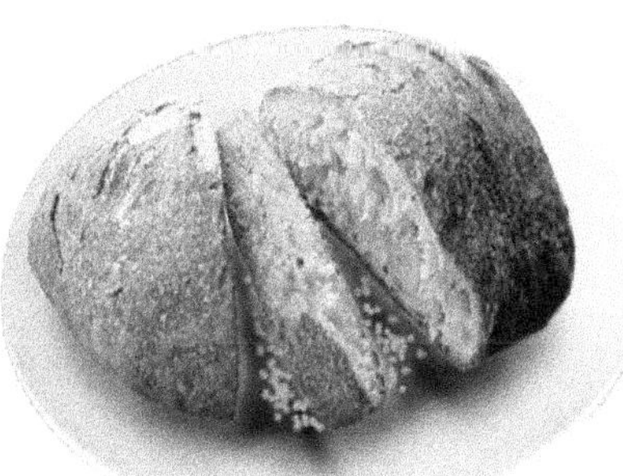

Eight or more of these chemicals are commonly used, including high salt. Did you know, for instance, that gelatine is one possible ingredient? It is produced from animal skin and bones. And of course, if you eat white bread, the flour has been bleached and stripped of its fibre and vitamins. Bleaching agents such as potassium bromate, azodicarbonamide, or chlorine dioxide are used. And then there is L-Cysteine, which is an amino acid - used as a flour improver.

L-Cysteine is permitted in all biscuits, bread and cakes, except those that claim to be wholemeal. L-Cysteine is produced from chicken or goose feathers, pig bristles and even human hair, mainly coming from China. The hair is dissolved in acid and L-cysteine is isolated through a chemical process, then packaged and shipped off to commercial bread producers. It can be produced synthetically, by fermentation, utilizing a mutant of E. coli. This is, however, more expensive.

Other additives are fat and preservatives to prolong shelf life.

When the bread has been baked, additional fat is pumped into it, obviously increasing its calories.

Normally, home made bread takes several hours to make, but factory bread is made in half and hour. It is pumped with air and forced to rise, leaving the yeast partially fermented. When you eat this, it continues to ferment in your gut, causing bloating.

Bread machines are reasonably cheap and easy to use. We have been using one for years to produce delicious, wholesome bread, containing only six natural ingredients – wholemeal flour, butter, salt, sugar, yeast and water. The cost of the bread is less than shop bought bread and lasts up to three days – but it is usually eaten by then.

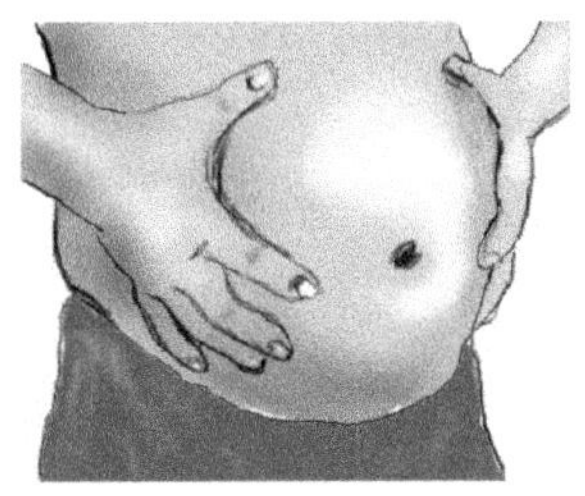

2(s). LOOK AFTER YOUR WAISTLINE

A spreading waistline could be a precursor to cancer, diabetes and heart disease

Middle age spread seems to be affecting us earlier and earlier these days. We see men who look as if they are eight months pregnant and laughingly call it a 'beer belly'. Women too seem to be spreading in that direction at a young age.

If you have a bulging waist you need to be concerned, because it is a precursor to diabetes and heart disease. If you are a woman, anything over about 31.5 inches or 80cm is too big. For men, a waist measurement of 37 inches (94 cm) or more might indicate a risk. You need to bear in you're your height and build as well, however. If you are very tall and muscular with a big bone structure, your measurements may be perfectly normal.

Fat around the waist indicates that you are storing internal fat. It may well be around your internal organs, as well as under your belly. This type of fat is difficult to shift. The first thing you need to do is stop eating junk food and ready meals and take control of what you are eating. You don't need to live on lettuce leaves – just eat smaller portions, eat slowly and eat healthily.

If you really want to lose weight, and you don't fancy joining a diet group, I recommend you try hypnosis. Hypnosis cannot make you do anything you don't want to and it is very relaxing. There are plenty of books and CD's out there.

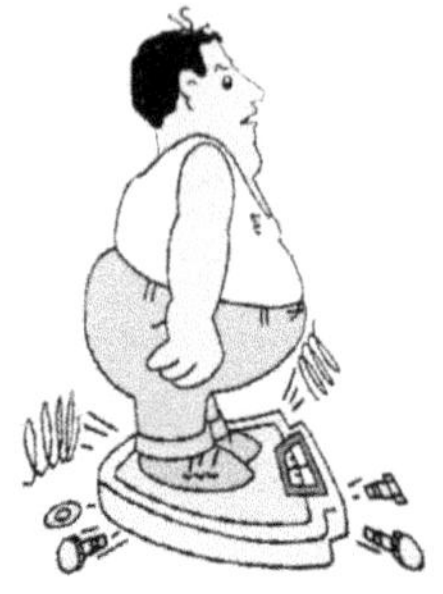

2(t). WHY DIETS DON'T WORK

Dieting can ultimately make you gain weight

Before you get upset by this statement, I will qualify it – diets don't work ... unless you change your eating habits forever. If you decrease your calorie input and increase your exercise, you will lose weight, provided that your calorie *output* is more than your calorie *input.*

Have you noticed that people lose weight from their heads downwards? The face and neck seem to slim down first, followed by the chest area. Fat on the tummy and hips is usually reluctant to go – we have different types of fat and the serious hoarding type is situated here in women and on the belly in men.

The diet and fitness industry is worth 6 billion pounds a year. If we all lost the weight and kept it off they would go bankrupt – but they are thriving. They come up with more and more ingenious diet plans to help us lose weight, knowing that once we have achieved our goal, we will go back to our old eating habits and put it all on again.

Our bodies also play a mean trick on us. We are born with a set-point, which dictates our rate of metabolism and keeps our bodies a healthy size. It governs our appetites and fat storage. However, when we starve we alter our set-point and our metabolism slows down. Then, when we return to normal eating our lowered set-point makes us conserve energy and therefore if we don't eat smaller portions, we will put on weight.

Some people resort to drastic measures. They have gastric surgery. They can either have a gastric band fitted, to decrease the stomach size, or have a gastric bypass, where a large part of the stomach is removed and a long section of intestine is cut out of the system. The remaining intestine is reconnected to the new walnut sized stomach. Weight loss is nearly always dramatic and as long as the patient eats very small meals forever, he or she will lose weight and keep it off. Some people cheat though and either eat plenty of calorie rich food, such as ice cream, or keep stuffing their tiny stomach until it stretches almost back to its original size.

If you are on a diet and are losing weight steadily you will need to reprogramme your body and mind. Eat healthy food, eat slowly, drink plenty of fluids and learn to recognise when you are hungry and when you are full. When you reach your target weight don't go back to the lifestyle that made you put on weight and remember that today is the first day of the rest of your life.

3. HYDRATION

Drinking the wrong things can definitely make you gain weight, or find it hard to shift it. Many processed drinks contain vast amounts of sugar and/or chemical additives. The body responds to chemicals by covering them in fat. Even if you are on a diet, drinking caffeine and aspartame laden drinks can make weight loss far more difficult.

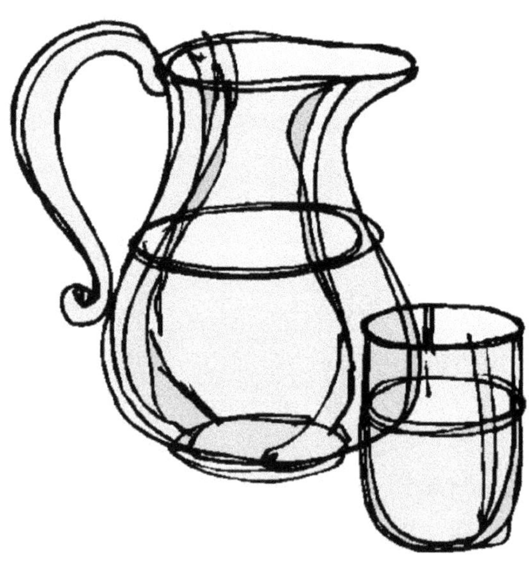

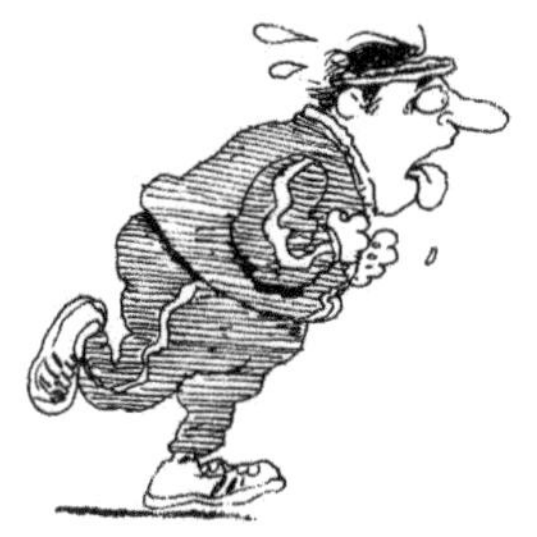

3(a). DRINK WHEN YOU ARE THIRSTY

Our bodies are 75% water and we need to drink regularly to enable the uptake of nutrients, elimination of waste and regulation of all the vital functions in our bodies. It is important that our blood maintains its liquidity in order for it to oxygenate our bodies, keep our internal organs working efficiently, keep our brain chemistry stable and enable us to fight bacterial and viral infections.

> *Long term body drought can precipitate chronic diseases*

If you weigh yourself, in the nude, just before you go to bed, and then again when you wake up, you should find your weight has decreased. Most of this is due to water loss. We positively leak water all the time – through our lungs, bodily fluids and sweat. If you put on a pair of rubber gloves for any length of time they will get wet. And if you breathe on glass it will be covered in condensation.

Some people say you should drink at least a litre of water a day. It depends on how much water there is in your food, how hot (or cold the weather is) and whether you are active or not. Some people sweat far more than others, anyway. Try to think about whether you are thirsty or not and let your body be your guide. Don't become obsessive about drinking water, though, if you drink too much you can affect the viscosity of your blood and deplete your body of electrolytes.

If you are a tea or coffee drinker you will need to drink more, because both contain caffeine, which is a stimulant. Caffeine stimulates the adrenal glands to release adrenaline, which in turn can either make you feel more awake, or jittery (adrenaline is the stress hormone). Caffeine can also affect you if you are diabetic because adrenaline is linked to the release of insulin and blood sugar.

The best time to drink is when you wake up in the morning. Your body is dehydrated and needs replenishing. Water is vital for maintaining healthy kidneys and blood viscosity. It keeps your lungs and digestive tract supple, as well as your skin and saliva in you mouth.

Many of us get dehydrated without even realising it. Drinking only pure water would be ideal but far from realistic. As long as there is a high percentage of water in your drink, it is OK but *don't* make a habit of drinking colas and other drinks with caffeine in them. And avoid drinks with high acidity and sweetness. Acid drinks, such as colas, dissolve the protective coating on your teeth and sugar turns to acid in your mouth, having the same effect. It also raises your blood sugar and can lead to diabetes. Cola is also addictive.

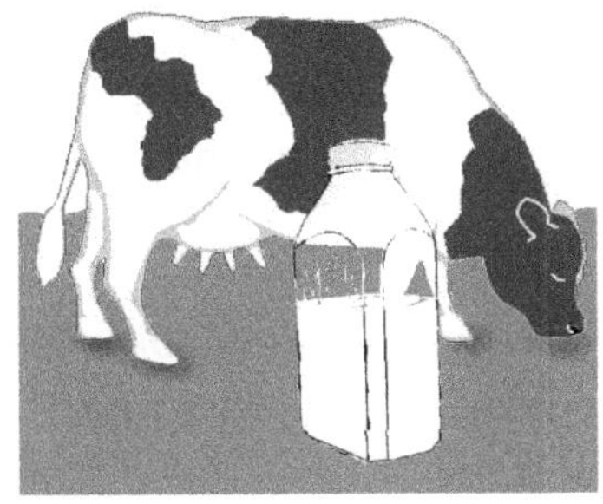

3(b).LIMIT YOUR MILK INTAKE

There is much controversy about milk. You may think it is the most basic of our staple foods and is really good for us. It is true that it contains proteins, vitamins and minerals but it was designed for baby cows, not humans. It is basically a food, not a drink and one cup contains 167 calories (full cream), 130 calories (reduced fat) or 110 calories (skimmed).

> Most milk contains titanium dioxide and permitted levels of puss

As babies we have our mother's milk to keep us alive. We possess a special milk-digesting enzyme specifically for human milk. This enzyme diminishes as we get older and in many people disappears altogether so they are unable to break down milk protein. Some lactose intolerant people can become extremely ill if they drink milk.

Others have vague symptoms such as asthma, eczema, skin rashes, stomach-ache, runny nose, diarrhoea ... Some people just never feel on form and don't know why.

Milk is a food, so obviously has far more calories than water. And Titanium Dioxide is added to make cows milk white – normally it is a bluish colour. In most industrially produced milk are permitted levels of puss. This is because intensively milked cows often have mastitis. There are also permitted levels of antibiotics and pesticides in milk. Large herds of cows have to be carefully managed and treated against diseases and pests.

Today's milk is normally homogenised – a process whereby the fat particles are forced into it so it doesn't separate. These tiny particles of fat can easily pass straight through the digestive tract without being broken down – a bit like having butter floating in your blood. Fat free milk is thin a watery, almost negating the reason for having it in the first place.

There are plenty of substitutes for cow's milk – rice milk, oat milk, almond milk, and soya milk. Soy is also used to make yoghurt – a good source of healthy bacteria for your gut.

Alcohol is addictive and can give you cancer, brain damage and liver disease

3(c). LIMIT YOUR ALCOHOL INTAKE

Alcohol is made from the fermentation of grains, fruits or vegetable matter. It starts with yeast or bacteria, which feed on sugars in the organic matter to produce ethanol and carbon dioxide.

It is the ethanol in alcohol which depresses your central nervous system, with a range of side-effects. Your cell membranes are highly permeable to alcohol and it quickly permeates into almost all your body tissues. If you have a heavy meal before drinking, the absorption rate will be slower, so drinking on an empty stomach is a recipe for disaster.

Hydration of the body and viscosity of the blood determines the body's ability to process alcohol. If you are dehydrated you are far more likely to experience a hangover after a heavy night's drinking. If alcohol consumption is too high, you can become unconscious and become a victim of alcohol poisoning - 0.4% is enough to kill you and if that doesn't get you, vomiting whilst unconscious can cause suffocation.

A drink's alcohol content is affected by how long it's left to ferment and spirits are distilled, removing the water and leaving a stronger concentration of alcohol.

Alcohol is addictive and if you drink large amounts regularly you will damage your liver and brain. Brain scans of heavy drinkers show patterns of 'holes' in the brain similar to those caused by Alzheimer's disease. Liver damage is life threatening. The liver performs many vital functions and one of it main jobs is to break down toxins. Over consumption of alcohol over extended periods damages the liver so it can no longer function. Alcohol is a psychoactive toxin that increases our risk of cancer, dementia as well as liver disease.

A few years ago I watched a friend slowly dying from alcoholism. Ironically he had 'dried out' and hadn't drunk for some time, but his liver was so badly damaged he had a prolonged and painful death.

On the positive side, regularly consuming a small amount of red wine appears to be good for you – it can even help you to live longer. It is thought that the antioxidants and resveratrol in red wine protect the cardiovascular system, reduces blood pressure and increases HDL cholesterol.

On the negative side, it is the ingredients of red wine, *minus* the alcohol that is good for you. A recent study has shown that natural antioxidant compounds in red wine – not the alcohol – are good for your heart health. Drinking alcoholic red wine cancels out most of the beneficial effects.

The toxicity of alcohol is worsened because as it is broken down for elimination from the body it is metabolised to acetaldehyde, an even more toxic substance. If the food industry tried to market a food with the equivalent of one unit of alcohol amount of acetaldehyde that a unit of alcohol, it would be banned as having an unacceptable health risk.

So what is the recommended daily limit for sensible drinking? Well, according to Professor David Nutt, a public health specialist: 'the idea that drinking small amounts of alcohol will do you no harm is a myth'. The current recommendation for women is 2-3 units or less and for men 3-4 units or less. If you choose to drink when you're pregnant (or planning to become pregnant), you should consume no more than 1-2 units of alcohol once or twice a week.

A unit of alcohol is half a pint of ordinary strength lager/beer/cider (3.5% ABV)

OR

25 ml pub measure of spirit (40% ABV)

OR

A small glass of wine (9% ABV)

4. HOMEOSTASIS

Enzymes only work at body temperature and are vital for our health

Homeostasis means keeping a constant internal environment. There are minimum of six functions which keep the body's organs operating efficiently. These are:

a. Carbon dioxide - it is in the air we breathe, we extract the oxygen and exhale carbon dioxide and other gases. If we are unable to regulate carbon dioxide the body becomes too acidic.

b. Urea - the waste produced by digesting amino acids (protein) in the liver. It is mainly eliminated in the urine but is also a component of sweat.

c. Ions - These are atoms or molecules that have gained (negative) or lost an electron (positive). They control the take-up and release of nutrients and waste products. If the balance of ions is not right, our cells can become dehydrated or over hydrated, leading to cell death. Important ions include sodium, potassium, hydrogen and phosphate. These are controlled through our urine and the amount of water we drink. We also lose some, like sodium ions, through our faeces and our sweat.

d. Sugar – blood glucose is essential to give us energy and without it we cannot survive.

e. Water - Seventy percent of our body mass is water. The kidneys are the main controller of fluids in the body, although some is eliminated through out lungs and skin.

f. Temperature - the enzymes that control every chemical reaction in our body work within a very narrow temperature range. If our body cells get too hot or too cold they would die.

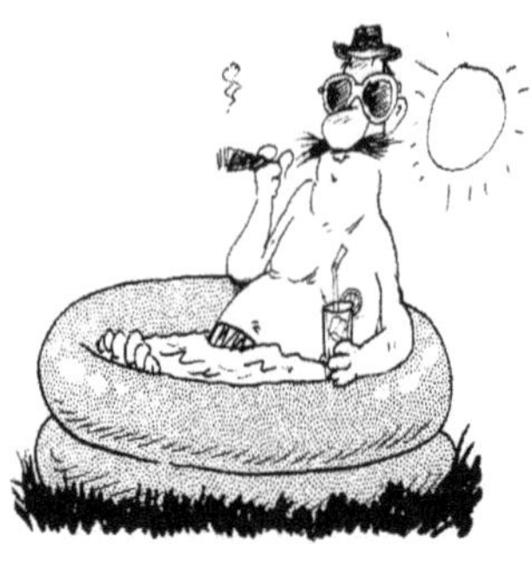

4(a). TRY TO MAINTAIN AN EVEN BODY TEMPERATURE

Our bodies are very smart at maintaining an even temperature, usually between 36.5 and 38 degrees centigrade (37.5 is the ideal). This constancy is called homeostasis. We need to maintain an even temperature because we have many enzymes in our bodies that only work in this narrow range. Incidentally, the enzymes in biological washing powders also need these temperatures to break down organic dirt in our clothes.

If our body temperature drops, the enzymes cannot perform the chemical reactions in our bodies fast enough to sustain life. Catalase is an enzyme that exists in almost all living organisms that breathe oxygen. Its job is to aid the decomposition of hydrogen peroxide into water and oxygen.

If the body temperature increases above that, the enzymes will start to denature and can no longer perform their chemical reactions.

It is only because we live in a sheltered environment and wear clothes that we have been able to migrate all around the world. Our ancient cousins, the apes, are unable to protect themselves from bad weather, although they do make 'umbrellas' from overhead leafy branches and huddle up, so they obviously dislike the rain as much as we do, because it makes them cold.

Newborn babies are very vulnerable to heat loss, as their temperature control is not fully functional. We instinctively wrap them up to protect them against hypothermia. Elderly people too, become victims of the cold. As we get older, we lose our sensitivity to cold and if we are hard up, we can't afford to keep our homes adequately heated in the winter. If you or an elderly relative are struggling to keep warm, wear several layers of clothing, keep one room warm, and have plenty of hot drinks and meals. If I am cold, and I am sedentary (writing books) I heat a wheat bag in the microwave and put it around my neck or under my clothing, ensuring it is not too hot.

Wearing a hat, even though you have a good head of hair, is also beneficial as heat rises and our heads are prone to heat loss, because there is a large skin surface on our faces and necks. Heat escapes quickly in cold weather, so if you can, exercise to keep yourself warm.

Hyperthermia, or overheating, is also life-threatening. Not only is hot weather a threat, but also developing a fever from an infection. The body deliberately raises its core temperature in order to kill the invading organisms. But if the temperature goes too high, it will kill. Sweating is our body's way of reducing our temperature. It evaporates on our skin, having a cooling effect. But if we wear clothes, there is nowhere for the sweat to go, so we remain hot and get smelly.

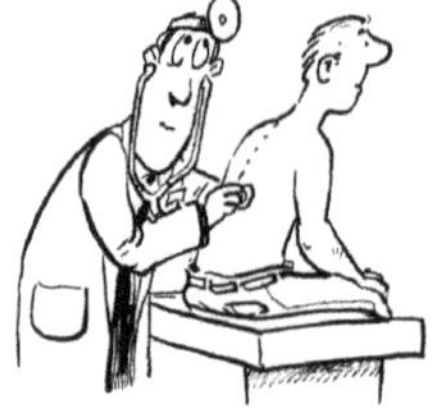

4(b). HAVE AN ANNUAL HEALTH CHECK

Having a regular health check could save your life

I have often thought that everyone, if possible, should have an annual health check. In the UK we have to health check our cars every year (MOT) so why don't we catch impending illnesses early, rather than treat them, when it is too late?

I discussed this with my friends and family and they all agree they would be happy to pay for the reassurance of a bona fide health check. And obviously, if people can't afford it, they should be able to get one for free.

There are several companies that offer routine health checks. We go to our local supermarket, where their pharmacy does an annual check for a very reasonable amount. The results of this showed raised blood pressure with my husband and raised cholesterol with me. However, once I had my cholesterol levels checked for LDL and HDL, it was found that I have a higher than average amount of low density lipoproteins, which is healthy. I do eat a lot of oily food, so I was right to be worried – but as I have plenty of healthy HDL cholesterol I will stick to my oil rich diet and continue munching on nuts every day, it keeps me fit and healthy.

A basic health checks monitors your blood pressure, blood sugar, weight, and body mass index.

High blood pressure indicates a constriction in the arterial system, resulting in potential blockages, heart attacks or strokes.

High blood sugar points to diabetes or pre-diabetes, where the pancreas is failing to produce enough insulin to deal with your blood glucose, or you have become insulin resistant. Late onset diabetes (type 2) is treatable with Metformin in the early stages or insulin injections when that no longer works. It is a condition to avoid if at all possible as the long term health prospects are not good, especially if you don't change your diet, lose weight and manage your illness carefully.

Monitoring your weight is valuable because carrying excess weight can cause diabetes, heart problems and cancer. It also puts an extra strain on your joints, can cause hiatus hernia and make you susceptible to yeast and skin infections, especially if you have folds of overhanging skin, which get hot and sweaty.

Body mass index indicates the amount of internal fat you have inside your body. You may not have much on the outside but if you have a significant amount around your internal organs you are far more likely to develop heart disease or diabetes. A BMI of over 25 is an indication that you are carrying too much internal fat.

In an ideal world we should also have a full body scan. This would show bone density and any potential early growths or tumours, as well as internal fat. MRI scans are very expensive. I hope that in the future someone will invent a cheap machine that can scan and monitor safely – it would save the lives of thousands.

Beware of companies which bombard you with literature or cold call you – many of them charge a fortune and give you exaggerated or inaccurate results, making you feel scared and encouraging you to spend even more money on further tests.

Eating and drinking from plastic bottles and packaging, could cause cancer

4(c). CHECK YOUR BREASTS REGULARLY

Breast cancer kills thousands of people a year and is a rising epidemic. This is thought to be caused by changes in the body caused by pollution, damaged trans-fats, smoking, drinking alcohol, obesity and unhealthy lifestyles. In these instances, homeostasis fails to protect us from cancerous growths. Taking the contraceptive pill also carries a slight risk of breast cancer. Some families have a much higher genetic risk and in this case some women opt to have a mastectomy. Men, too can develop breast cancer, although it is much rarer.

During your fertile years it is important to examine your breasts one a month, just after a period when they are at their least lumpy. There are plenty of places where you can find out the best way for self-examination – a good description can be found on: www.breastcancer.org/symptoms/testing/types/self_exam/bse_steps

It is common for women to have tender breasts during their childbearing years and often they are lumpy too. If you examine them every month you may be able to feel if anything has changed. Even if you do find a lump it will probably be harmless but always check if you find one.

Older women in the UK are offered breast screening, where each breast is clamped between two plates and an x-ray taken, from different angles. There is some controversy over this, as the x-rays (and potential bruising of breast tissue) carry a small risk. However the risk is nowhere near as high as the risk of ignoring sinister breast lumps.

To minimise the chances of breast cancer you should stop smoking, cut out alcohol and avoid trans-fats (hydrogenated fats). When eaten frequently hydrogenated fats are used by the body to make up cell membranes and fat cells. As the breasts contain fat and tissue which is subject to constant hormonal changes, they are more prone to cancerous growths.

There is some evidence to show that plastic food containers can leach chemicals if they are scratched or heated. It is also likely that frequent exposure to some of these chemicals, such as bisphenol A (BPA), could cause cancer in people. For this reason, never leave a plastic bottle of drink in a car or other hot place, especially if the sun is shining on it. Nor should you heat food in rigid plastic containers in the microwave.

A variety of chemicals including BPA, which are found in many rigid plastics, can linings, dental sealants and paper till receipts, act as a week oestrogen and become a hormone disruptor. These synthetic hormones can affect how oestrogen and other hormones act in the body, by blocking them or mimicking them. This disrupts the body's hormonal balance.

Here is another alarming revelation. BPA is also thought to affect brain development of unborn babies. A study has recently shown that pregnant women with high levels of BPA in their urine were more likely to have daughters who develop hyperactivity, anxiety, and depression. These symptoms became apparent in girls as young as 3. Boys do not seem to be affected in the same way.

Using tanning beds before the age of 30 can increase your risk of skin cancer by 75%.

4(d). BEWARE OF SKIN DAMAGE FROM ULTRAVIOLET RAYS

Many of us enjoy sun bathing. It feels good to lie in the warmth of the sun and get a healthy tan. However, the evidence is now irrefutable that there are parts of the sun's spectrum of light that damage our skin and can cause cancer, sometimes a lot later on in our lives.

The dangers from the sun have increased steadily over recent years. Chemicals and fumes from factories and domestic appliances have been responsible for the hole in the ozone layer and it is also getting thinner. Chlorofluorocarbons (CFCs) used to be used in refrigerators but were found to be the main culprit for the ozone damage.

Unfortunately, more harmful sun's rays are now able to get through and damage our skins but did you know that there are two categories of harmful rays – UVA and UVB?

UVA rays shine constantly during daylight, no matter what season or climate so you can get sun damage on a cold, cloudy day. They penetrate through glass and even some clothing. Car drivers often have more skin damage on the arm next to the car door.

UVA rays used to be considered relatively safe and are widely used in tanning beds. However, it is now known that using tanning beds before the age of 30 can actually increase your risk of skin cancer by 75%.

UVA rays are responsible for the signs of ageing because they penetrate the surface of the skin, damaging the cells beneath.

UVB Rays are the ones which burn your skin. They are far stronger in the summer months but can also reflect off of water or snow. They are responsible for causing most skin cancers. While large doses of UVA rays can contribute to cancer, it's the UVB rays that are commonly to blame.

Obviously, know what we do about UV light, we need to protect our skins from the sun's rays. This particularly applies to children. It is no longer safe to allow them to play unprotected in the sun. Even if they appear to be OK now, they could be affected in the future.

When buying sunscreen lotions, go for those that specifically say UVA/UVB or "broad spectrum coverage" on the bottle. Sun protection factor (SPF) 15 is the minimum strength you should use and it should be reapplied every hour or two. To estimate the affectivity of your sunscreen, take the SPF number and multiply it by 10. That is the length of time you'd be safe from the sun's rays. So SPF 15 should last about 150 minutes, provided you don't wash or rub it off in the meantime.

5 SOMNOLENCE

'Sleep, that knits up the ravelled sleeve of care' - Shakespeare

Sleep is the time when your body repairs itself. Your heart and breathing rate reduce significantly and during this time of physical inactivity your body has a chance to make new cells, clear away detritus and return to a state of homeostasis - the maintenance of a more or less constant internal environment.

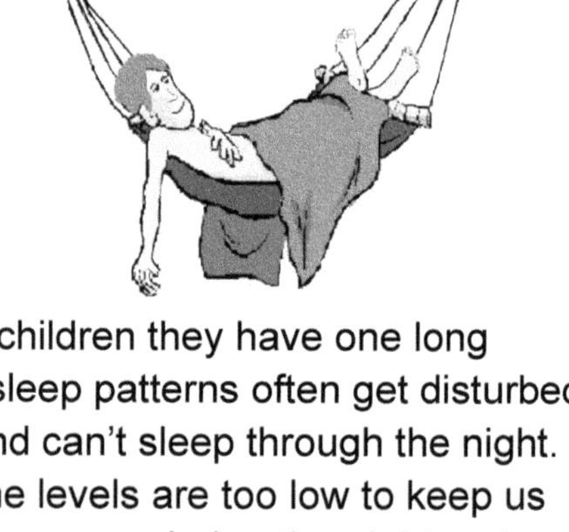

Different people need different amounts of sleep and young children need far more than adults. Babies start with poly-phasic sleep, where they sleep almost from feed to feed, until as children they have one long sleep a day. As we get older our sleep patterns often get disturbed and we find we doze in the day and can't sleep through the night. This is because our sleep hormone levels are too low to keep us asleep. If you are awake for an hour or so during the night and then go back to sleep, you often find it difficult to wake up and get going. Every time you go to sleep, a sleep hormone is released and so two periods of sleep close together results in higher hormone levels than normal. This hormone is broken down by the liver, to enable you feel wide awake.

Our lives are governed by a circadian body clock, which is located deep in our brains. It is set by the earth's day and night cycle. I remember, years ago, seeing an experiment with a group of people who agreed to live in isolation, with no natural daylight and no contact with the rest of the world. They slept when they were tired and ate when they were hungry.

It was found that their natural body clocks gradually adjusted until their days were about an hour shorter than normal – they had a 23 hour routine. This puzzled the researchers for some time until they realised that the spinning of our planet is gradually slowing down and when our far distant ancestors were evolving, the days were shorter.

As we approach our usual sleep time our body clocks start to slow down the functions in our bodies to help prepare us for the night of sleep. In this way we can go hours without food or water, although we may be disturbed in the night to go to the toilet. In the darkness of night, we secrete a hormone called melatonin, to promote sleepiness. It suppresses itself during daylight to keep us awake. If you are a shift worker and have to sleep during the day, you often don't get the good quality sleep that you need. Even when people are used to night work, they experience a dip at about three in the morning, when they feel tired and less able to concentrate.

Sleep is vital, not only for body repair but also for a healthy state of mind. There are two different types of sleep – rapid eye movement (REM) sleep and NREM (non-rapid eye movement). During REM we dream and this seems to be the brain's way of unscrambling the thousands of signals it receives and transmits each day. When we remember a dream we can often relate parts of the dream to things that have happened, or things that have been said, either recently or in the past. However, our dreams get jumbled up into bizarre imagined events and often reflect things that we are worrying about or frustrations we are trying to deal with.

Sleep deprivation was, and probably still is, used to torture people. If you go days without sleep your mind will start wandering and you will have visions and dreams, even though you are still awake.

If you travel to another part of the world your body clock will be disturbed. Known as 'jet-lag', you feel awful. You can't concentrate, you feel physically drained and you can't sleep when you're supposed to. It takes two to three days for you to adjust to the new time zone.

If you are having trouble sleeping, try sticking to a set routine, telling your subconscious mind that bedtime is coming. If you are stressed try having a soak in the bath, with a few drops of lavender in the water, and a bedtime drink (but not caffeine). Ensure your bedding is warm (or cool) enough and comfortable. Put up heavy curtains if street lights disturb you. You might enjoy a good read, or to watch TV in bed – anything to stop you thinking your own thoughts.

Another strategy is to put on a meditation CD or even a self-hypnosis CD. Hypnosis is perfectly safe – you will never do anything your conscious mind doesn't want you to do. Deep breathing can make you relaxed, especially if you have to concentrate on timed breath holding and releasing.

If my mind is too busy to allow me to sleep I try to picture things in my mind in all the colours of the rainbow. So I picture, say, a red rabbit and gradually turn it orange, yellow, etc. It usually works – sometimes I manage to picture beautiful patterns and lights – I find it fascinating.

In order to sleep well you need to have enough food in your stomach, so you aren't hungry. Conversely, if your stomach is too full, it will stop you dozing off.

6. TOUCH

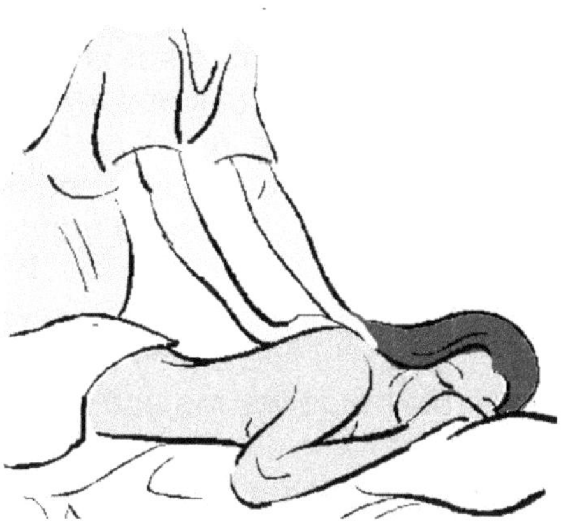

Human touch is essential for physical and mental well-being

Years ago I saw a television programme which deeply moved me and which I will never forget. It was about the importance of touch and involved two baby monkeys. They were both deprived of their mothers. One was given a surrogate mother in the form of a fur-covered object and the other had nothing. The poor little animal with nothing cowered in the corner of its cage, and became emotionally disturbed. The monkey with the furry surrogate spent all its time clinging to its 'mother', reluctant to leave it, even to feed. It did, however, fair better than the other one.

Human touch (and interaction) are vital for our emotional development. It is a well-known fact that people who have grown up in regimented children's homes or were starved of affection, became emotionally unbalanced. Some developed criminal tendencies, some became very depressed, some were full of self loathing and some physically harmed themselves.

As parents, most of us instinctively cuddle our babies and children. And if we don't have a baby to cuddle, we'll cuddle a dog, cat, or even soft toys. Humans are very tactile – they shake hands when they meet someone (so do chimps), they put a hand on someone's shoulder when they are upset, and they kiss people when they greet. In some countries it is considered insulting not to embrace someone when you first meet.

Years ago I went through a bout of back trouble, most of which was caused by stress. I finally went to see an osteopath. I had seen many other practitioners but this one was different. She was cheerful and caring and used heat lamps and massage to soothe my protesting muscles before she manipulated my body. I was so impressed with the effects of the massage that I decided to train as a massage therapist.

I am still practising those skills and all my patients come to me for pain and stress relief. Massage warms and oxygenates the muscles and helps to remove irritating waste products from the nerves and tissues. I have continued my education over the years and hope that I now have a fair bit of expertise in the field of therapeutic massage.

I really enjoy what I do – I find that working so closely with people, makes me feel relaxed and at one with myself. If your relationship is a bit stale, why not try more touching? With this in mind, I wrote 'Romantic Massage' (ISBN-10: 1477551123 or ISBN-13: 978-1477551127). This book gives step by step instructions for several different types of massage, as well as the use of essential oils and the benefits of massage on the body.

If you are deprived of touch I recommend you have a massage, improve your own relationship, find someone to love or get a pet. Whatever you do, touch is vital, and especially for children. Without touch from an early age we become depressed and anti-social.

7. PHYSICAL AND MENTAL STIMULATION

Early stimulation of the mind lights the spark to a creative future

One of the reasons why man has become so dominant in the world is because of his never-ending ability to go beyond his natural boundaries. People can live in almost any part of the world by adapting to their environment. Most animals need stimulus – the more intelligent they are, the more they need. I was watching a group of dolphins recently, playing with a fallen branch in the water. They were playing all sorts of games with it, passing it to each other, circling round it and chasing each other for it. This behaviour had nothing to do with catching food, it was pure mental stimulation.

I have also seen amazing experiments with chimps, where they proved they could recall long sequences of objects, in the right order, by touching a screen – they were far quicker, and hard far better memories, than their human keepers. Chimps can also learn sign language and use it to convey their thoughts to others. It is our ability to form our thoughts into complex language that makes us different from the rest of the animal kingdom. It is true that animals have their own language for communicating with each other, but it is nowhere near as sophisticated as ours.

By speaking, recording, drawing and writing things down we have been able to pass on everything we learn, forming a vast database of knowledge available to the rest of the human race to share. So instead of just learning things that our families teach us, we learn from the rest of the world as well.

Our brains are far bigger (in proportion to the rest of our bodies) than other animals. Throughout our evolution we have become extremely clever and the more clever we become, the more we want to know.

We instinctively stimulate babies. We hold them at their natural range of focus (about 25cm away from our faces) and talk to them, looking into their eyes to ensure we have their full attention. It doesn't matter what we say at first, it's the tone of voice that counts. Even before they are born they can hear their mother's voice and they are already learning about language and emotions. It isn't long before a baby will start exploring its environment, first with its mouth and hands and later using all its senses. Most babies are given toys – noisy toys, soft toys, brightly coloured toys. We instinctively know that they need stimulation to help them to develop.

As we grow older, most of us go to school. We are bombarded with new facts all day and every day and gradually we amass a huge amount of knowledge. Children up to the age of four have brains like sponges – then is the time to stretch their potential. I have seen babies able to recognize words and communicate with sign language. The more you stimulate a child's mind, the more self confident and well socialised they will become. Children who receive plenty of stimuli when they are young, grow into intelligent and confident adults. These people are the leaders of tomorrow.

Many people who live with very little stimulation become bored, dull and depressed. We are fortunate to have televisions and computers, which go some way to solving the problem. Books are also a good way to stimulate the mind. Solitary confinement is one of the cruelest modes of torture, it can turn us insane. Many people are lonely and isolated. They spend their lives on their own, with no-one to talk to or share things with. This leads to misery and depression. If you know of someone who is lonely, try paying them a visit, it might change their lives for the better.

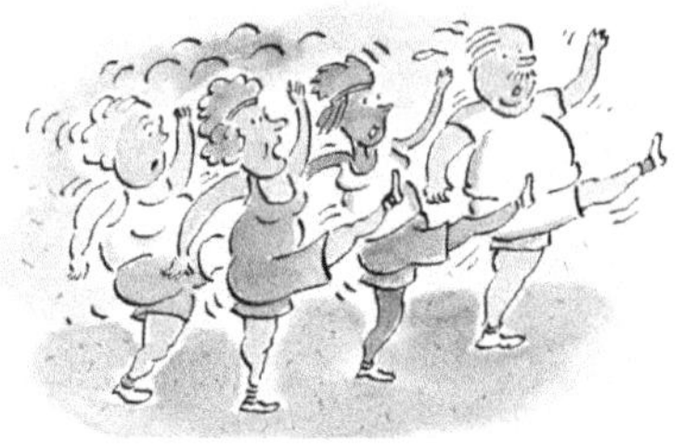

7(a). EXERCISE REGULARLY

Exercise keeps you healthy and makes you feel good

The human race has evolved to be active (unlike the sloth or panda). Coming from ancestors who were tree climbers and long distance walkers, we are equipped with a flexible spine and four limbs to help us to move around, finding food or running away from predators.

Our muscles are made up of packages of stretchy fibrous material. Every fibre of the muscle is made up of a number of very thin strands called fibrils. One square centimetre of muscle contains up to one million fibres. Each fibre has its own nerve, which makes it contract. It is the number of contracting fibres that determines the strength of a muscle.

Our muscles also have a vast supply of blood capillaries, which get squeezed and stimulated every time we use them. The more we exercise, the more muscle we grow and therefore the more blood supply we develop. Muscles actually generate heat, so if our muscles are well toned it will help to keep us warm. Muscles also help the blood to circulate around our bodies, especially the calf muscles, which squeeze slow moving blood back to the heart, when we walk, lessening the risk of varicose veins.

Exercise is good for us, but we don't necessarily have to go to the gym. In fact evidence shows that vigorous exercise for extended period is bad for us. Exercise increases our heart and breathing rates, helping our bodies to eliminate carbon dioxide from our lungs and potential arterial narrowing plaque from our circulatory systems. The Government are currently advocating 150 minutes of exercise a week, but only about 38% of men and 28% of women meeting those targets.

Another benefit of exercise is that it makes us feel good. How many times have you gone for a walk to clear your head? Walking oxygenates the body, and in particular the brain.

Exercise has been shown to reduce stress and its associated aches and pains. As a therapist I regularly treat stress related disorders. Most of my patients spend hours at their computers and I always recommend that they try to get out and about more, moving their arms around to lubricate their joints and maybe even join an exercise group.

When we exercise, our levels of the stress hormone, cortisol, reduces and the feel-good hormones, the endorphins increase. When endorphins are released they boost our mood. Exercise also releases adrenaline, serotonin, and dopamine. These chemicals work together to make you feel good

Endorphins are hormone-like substances that are produced in the brain. They are the body's natural painkillers. During exercise, these endorphins are released, and this can produce feelings of euphoria and a general state of well-being. The endorphins produced can be so powerful that they actually mask pain. Physically active people recover from mild depression more quickly and physical activity is strongly correlated with good mental health as people age.

Exercise builds muscle and lubricates your joints, stimulates your digestive system, increases blood flow and oxygenates the body, so what is stopping us from doing it?
The world of work dominates the lives of many of us. We spend hours at computers, machinery, desks or just sitting. Then when we get home we feel stressed and tired. All we

want to do is sit and relax. It actually takes exercise to motivate us to move around more. In fact some long distance joggers and cyclists are actually addicted to the feel-good hormones.

Have you ever come back from a walk and found that you are then motivated to cut the grass, or clean the car? You need to bite the bullet and just get up and move, even though you don't want to. I have a small trampoline, which I bought to get some exercise. However, it sits in the garden shed, unused for weeks on end because I won't make the time to use it – I am as guilty as everyone else, of making excuses.

When the weather is bad I move around indoors, vigorously cleaning the carpets or washing the floors. Failing that I will jog around the perimeter of the kitchen, especially if I am waiting for something to cook. I'll go ten laps in one direction and then ten the other, just to get out of breath and get my circulation flowing. I'm sure my family think I'm barmy but I don't care.

Boredom is a huge exercise de-motivator, which is why people sign up for a year's gym membership and then stop going. You need to be really sporty or have grim determination to exercise regularly, for health reasons. Having a lively dog can be a great excuse for walking. Having young children will also keep you fit. If you can, walk up stairs rather than take the lift, walk shorter distances, rather than drive the car and make a conscious effort to go for a walk at least once a day - you will be doing a lot to improve you muscle tone and general fitness.

I bought a blood pressure monitor some time ago and decided to monitor my blood pressure and also my husband's. I was concerned to see his blood pressure was bordering on being too high. He immediately did something about it – he went out for an early morning strenuous walk, every day. That was fine while the weather was good but when it came to winter he lost his motivation. His blood pressure is now rising again.

There are four main types of exercise – low impact, aerobic, high intensity and low intensity. All have their benefits but some are better than others.

Low impact exercises, such as swimming, pilates and yoga are excellent for stretching your muscles and building up strength. Yoga should involve breathing techniques as well, which oxygenates the lungs. If you are overweight or suffering from arthritis these may help. Failing that, try and do whatever you can to move regularly, challenging yourself to do a little more each day. You should find that as you get stronger you are more able to cope with your physical and emotional problems.

Aerobic exercises are prolonged high-energy exercises which force more oxygen into the bloodstream and tissues. They are quite often done to music and can be fun, especially if you go to an aerobics class. I wouldn't recommend aerobics to anyone who has been sedentary for some time. It is best to build up your exercise gradually to avoid strains and other injuries. In all cases of exercise you should warm your muscles first by gentle stretches and walking.

High intensity training (HIT) is making the headlines at the moment because it has been found to be very beneficial for reducing blood pressure. HIT consists of a batch of three short but intense workouts, with rests or low intensity exercise in between. Its benefits include an increase in aerobic capacity, carbohydrate metabolism and insulin sensitivity so it could help overweight diabetics as well as marathon runners.

You will need an exercise bike or trampoline or you could even run for 30-second bursts. Between each burst comes a four-minutes rest, or easy pedalling or walking. This needs to be repeated four to six times, three days a week.

Six weeks of HIT is equivalent to 20 weeks of traditional endurance training and sedentary men were found to have reductions in both glucose and insulin levels. However, is there any scientific evidence that the short-lived discomfort of HIT is an acceptable payoff for the time and effort of normal exercising you save? If you are very unfit it could cause you harm – it would be far better to start off gently and then give HIT a try when you are fitter.

Low intensity exercise would be something like ballroom dancing, walking or swimming a few lengths in the pool. It doesn't put any strain on your joints but does exercise your muscles and increases your pulse and breathing rates.

Jogging has become more popular lately and we often see people running along, with a water bottle in one hand and a cloth in the other to mop their sweaty brows. Unfortunately there are more running based injuries now than ever before. Constantly pounding your knee joints wears them out. The cartilage wears and exposes the bone. Cartilage is irreplaceable and the only solution is a knee replacement. The wrong shaped heel on your trainers can cause knee injuries as it alters the natural gait of a runner. If you buy trainers for running always make sure they are comfortable, flexible and low profile.

Whatever exercise you may choose to do, if it hurts, stop. There is bound to be some discomfort, a burning sensation in the muscles, but sharp pain is a clear indication to stop.

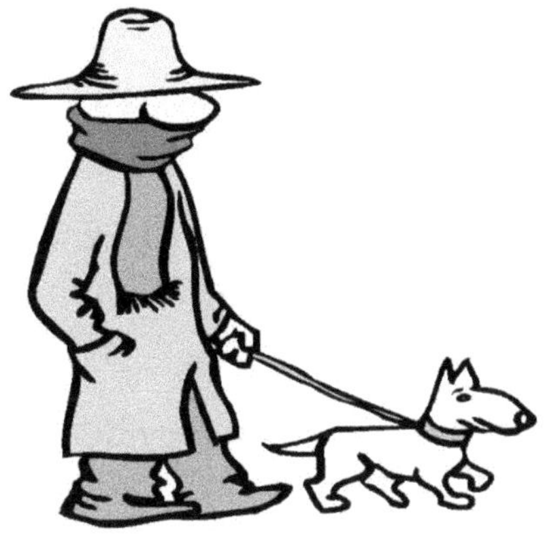

7(b). WALK, DON'T RUN

Frequent jogging can age your joints by up to 20 years

We have evolved over millions of years to do plenty of walking while we search for our food and take it back to our tribes. We are the only mammal that walks naturally on two legs with a straight spine and looking forward. Our pelvises have changed shape, and our leg bones have got thicker and longer. When we walk, we transfer all our weight from one leg to the other, so our two legs have to be as strong as our four legged friends.

Walking at a steady pace has several beneficial effects on our bodies. Our calf muscles squeeze the blood vessels in our legs and push the blood, against gravity, back to our hearts. The steady motion encourages our digestive systems to work efficiently, enabling us to have a healthy gut.

Walking raises our heart and breathing rate and increases the oxygen saturation in our bodies. It encourages the flow of lymph around our bodies and also perspiration, which is a means of eliminating some waste products. Gentle exercise is stimulating and encourages the release of endorphins, making us feel better. Regular walking also increases bone density and muscle tone.

One pound of body fat is equal to 3500 calories, and walking uses approximately 100 calories a mile, according to how much effort is involved. If you make the effort to walk regularly it could help you to lose weight and it will certainly tone your muscles.

Some people are natural runners. They have heaps of energy and they feel driven to run. However conditions are far different now from when we travelled over the African plains.

For a start we wear shoes, enclosing our feet so they don't flex naturally and take the force of each step. When we pound the roads and pavements in our trainers we are putting a lot of shock on our hip, knee and ankle joints. True, we have cartilage to enable the ends of the bones to slide on each other, but this eventually gets worn out, thus exposing the ends of our bones. This is very painful and causes arthritis.

Another problem with many trainers is that their soles are stiff and the heels are built up. When we run barefoot, the soles of our feet are the first to touch the earth, which yields under each footfall. Wearing trainers for running can damage our knees because of the faulty running action. Running regularly for prolonged periods can age your joints a good ten to twenty years.

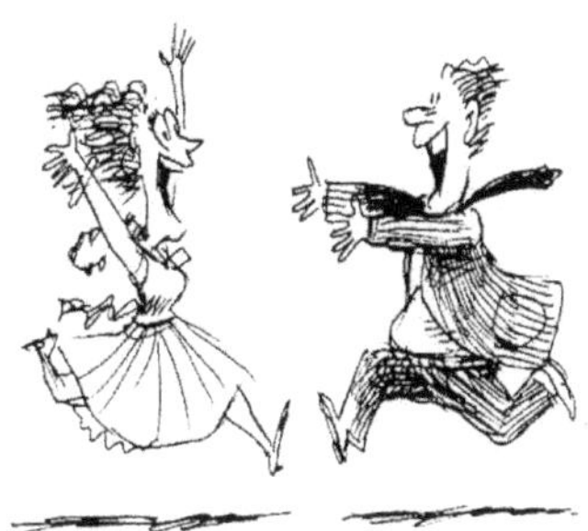

7c. BE SOCIABLE

Loneliness can make you ill

Humans are tribal, gregarious beings – they depend upon each other to survive. If a young child grows up without affection and friendship, he will develop depression and behavioural problems. Not many people are happy to always be on their own, although there are some.

We need friends and family and sometimes our friends are even more important than family because as the saying goes 'we can't choose our family but we can choose our friends'. Friends and colleagues are sounding boards for our thoughts and feelings and they make us feel needed. Loneliness can shorten our lives and send us into a downward spiral of misery.

If you are lonely try to find a group of people with similar interests to you. Maybe you're sporty, like singing, play bowls, enjoy painting ... there are so many things you could do. If you don't have any particular interests in life how do you spend your time? Do you devote yourself to your job? Or are you retired with nowhere to go and nothing to do all day? (If this is the case try to contact a local support group and get some help.)

Do yourself a favour and learn to be more sociable. I admit that if you are shy, joining groups is difficult. It is all to do with tribalism – you need to be accepted in someone else's tribe before you can feel at ease.

A second, though not ideal, option is to join an online group and get into some mind stimulating discussions. Whatever you do, be sociable and improve your self-esteem. Depression, anxiety, low self-esteem and stress can adversely affect your immune system and make you prone to infections.

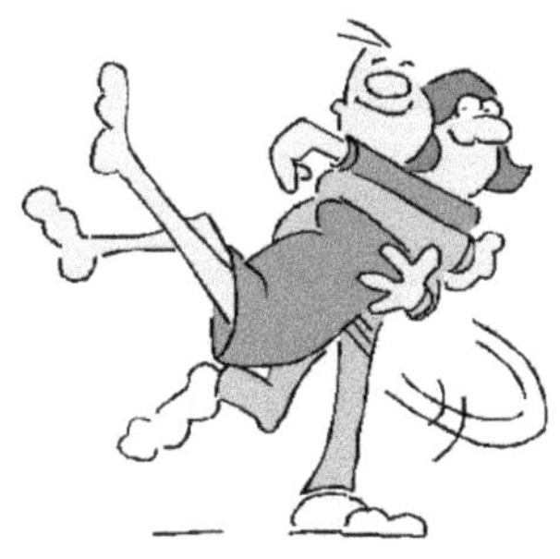

7(d.) WORK ON YOUR RELATIONSHIP OR FALL IN LOVE

> Semen contains hormones that can make a man's partner feel good

These days, about one in three marriages end in divorce and out of those divorced couples, half have children under sixteen. The majority of couples part in their early forties, often when the children are beginning to become independent and careers become more demanding. Having teenage children can put a huge strain on a relationship, as teenagers are often moody and challenging. However, young children can also put a strain on the marriage, as they are so demanding.

If you have spent years together, your relationship may well have gone stale. You get into a routine where there is very little quality time left to spend on each other. You take each other for granted and take out your frustrations on your partner. Apart from this there are temptations all around us from work colleagues and friends who seem attractive and attentive.

Divorce is very damaging, both emotionally and financially. It is particularly damaging to children – even the older ones feel hurt and guilty, wondering if they have caused the split. If you feel things are going wrong try your best to talk about it with your partner. Spicing up your love life could also help – try a few saucy DVD's, sexy underwear, toys or massage. And of course, spicing up your sex life can help too, especially if you don't use a condom.

Semen is the nutritious fluid that transports and nourishes sperm.

In fact, semen is a rich soup, containing testosterone, oestrogen, prostaglandins and also luteinizing hormone and follicle-stimulating hormone (which trigger ovulation). These chemicals are absorbed into a woman's bloodstream and can do much to improve her feel-good factor.

There are many marriage guidance organisations around, the hardest step is the first one – admitting (both of you) that you need help.

Falling in love is one of the best feelings. It makes us feel wanted, it improves our self esteem and raises our mood. If you are on your own I recommend it, despite the difficulties in finding a suitable partner. As we get older it is very difficult to find someone, especially if we don't socialise much. Joining a club or group may help, but most people tend there to already be in couples.

Dating agencies can be good if you can afford their fees. Failing that, internet dating is becoming very popular. The only problem is that people are not always honest and you could find yourself falling for someone who is already in a relationship, or who is not what they appear to be. Always meet in a public place, tell your friends where you are and allow plenty of time before committing yourself to someone.

Being independent helps you to cope through adversity

7(e). MAINTAIN YOUR INDEPENDENCE

It is great when you're in a really loving relationship and you do things for each other. When I was young it was accepted that there was 'men's work' and 'women's work'. A woman's place was doing the housework and looking after the home and a man's place was to be a wage earner and do all the manual jobs. However, I grew up in a home where both parents were handy with the tools. Despite being a girl, by the time I was twelve I was building my own rabbit hutches and tending the garden. Soon after that I re-decorated my bedroom and at sixteen I could service my motor bike.

I am eternally grateful to my parents for encouraging me to be independent. Whenever I asked my mother for help she would say 'God helps those who help themselves', so if I wanted something done I would do it myself.

This ability to fend for myself stood me in good stead when I suddenly found myself on my own, with a house to run. At that time, I remember a friend of mine being without a vacuum cleaner for over a year because she didn't know how to wire a plug (and her husband didn't care). I fixed the problem for her and she was eternally grateful. I think basic house maintenance should be taught in all schools and children should be encouraged to do more in the home.

Independence comes in many forms – from physical independence to financial independence. I had to learn about finance very quickly when my partner died and at first I really struggled. People can be over protective to their loved ones, preventing them from coping, should anything happen to them. When you are independent, you feel good about yourself because you don't have to keep asking for help. And of course if there is no one to help you, you can get really stuck, like my friend with her dustpan and brush.

Lack of independence can also be very expensive. There are many so-called 'experts' out there willing to rip you off for jobs you should be able to do for yourself. I once hired a plumber to take off a radiator, clean it out and replace it. He spent three hours on the job and charged me a fortune, as well as leaving the radiator leaking so I would have to call him back.

Another friend was completely dependent on her husband and his plans and wants. They did everything together, she had no hobbies or interests of her own and now he has died she is totally lost. She cries every day and can't wait to join him 'in heaven'. I know it is very sad to lose a loved one, it happened to me, but it is important that we make the best of what we have – my independence was the one thing that helped me to survive.

8. CLEANSING

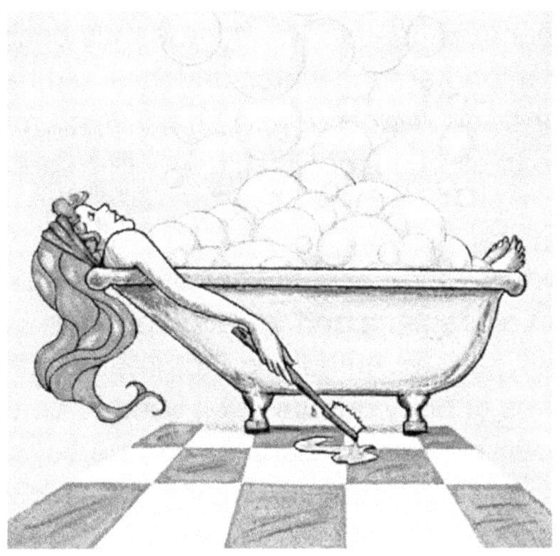

Skin is the largest organ of elimination in the body

Personal hygiene is very important. You have only to think of a baby and how much attention he needs. Every time he regurgitates his milk or soils his nappies we instinctively clean him. We know that if we didn't, his skin would very quickly become raw from yeast and bacterial infections.

Most of our problems stem from the fact that we have very little body hair and have to wear clothes to survive cold weather. This allows perspiration to dampen our clothes and skin and is an ideal place for bacteria and yeasts to grow and reproduce.

Our bodies clean themselves inside – dead matter and detritus is engulfed by specialist scavenger cells and eliminated from the body, with the help of our lymphatic system. We also sweat waste products through our skins. Sweat typically contains water, salt, vitamin C, antibodies, urea, uric acid, ammonia, and lactic acid. Sebum is produced by hair follicles to lubricate and protect the hair but it also accumulates on the skin, making it greasy and smelly.

I believe that humans need to wash frequently because they originally lived in and around water, which would have kept them clean. Great apes don't wash – apart from some monkeys in Japan who like to sit in hot pools all day – this keeps them warm in the winter.

If we don't wash we soon become smelly. This is because sweat is broken down by bacteria and yeasts, and their waste products cause the smell. Modern humans go to great lengths to cover up or rid themselves of body odours but it used to be thought sexy to have body odour. In the past, people used herbs, such as lavender, to disguise their smell. Thank goodness we now have soap and water!

Speaking of keeping clean, many children (and adults) don't wash their hands properly and bite their nails. This can cause parasitic infestations, mainly thread worms and sometimes tape worms. These feed on the food in their guts, robbing them of nutrients.

Did you know that 1 in 5 coffee cups in a typical busy office contain a killer virus – E. Coli? This bacterium comes from faecal matter. If people don't wash their hands after going to the toilet they spread E. Coli around the office. This can cause stomach upsets.

Many stomach upsets are caused by dirty dishcloths around the home. It is thought that more than a quarter of all household dishcloths are contaminated by the raw meat bacteria, E.Coli and around 14% harbour listeria. Soaking them in bleach or washing them by hand is no guarantee that they will be bacteria free. Boiling them for 15 minutes or putting them in your washing machine is the best way to kill the germs. Dishcloths should be changed every couple of days, and in any case, if your dishcloth smells, it's time to change it.

Women in particular have to pay particular attention to intimate hygiene. Accidentally wiping faecal matter from the back passage over the genitals can lead to cystitis. Bacteria travel along the short urethra and get into the bladder, where they cause infection. The symptoms are blood in the urine and a stinging and urgency during urination. Left untreated it can cause kidney infections and even blood poisoning.

Men also need to attend to intimate hygiene. Unless they are circumcised, a cheesy substance, called smegma builds up under the foreskin. It consists of stale lubricant oils exuded by the foreskin to allow it to slide over the glans, mixed with stale urine and semen plus shed skin cells and miscellaneous dirt and dust. It should be washed off with soapy water at least once a day to avoid bacterial infections and bad smells. Make sure the soap is completely washed off to avoid soreness.

It is a known fact that the incidence of cervical cancer, in the wives of circumcised men, is far less – perhaps indicating that male cleanliness is linked to female sexual health.

Keeping our teeth and mouths clean are also important. Other animals clean their teeth by eating high fibre raw foods. We accumulate plaque, mostly from food that sticks to our teeth. When plaque combines with acid it causes tooth decay.

Our tongues also harbour food particles in the rough papillae and mucous. Some foods, like milk and cheese encourage the growth of yeasts, giving the tongue a furry appearance and giving you bad breath. You can get tongue scrapers but I use my toothbrush, it seems to be just as effective. Flossing between the teeth removes particles of food that get lodged between them. Left unattended they rot and also cause bad breath. Visit your dentist regularly to keep you teeth and mouth healthy, brush your teeth regularly and use a mouth-wash.

Our noses cleanse themselves with mucous, which needs removing from time to time. Eyes also produce tear drops, and have lysosomes - cellular organelles - which produce natural antibiotics to keep the eyes healthy. Eyes need to be rinsed with clean water at least once a day.

Ears produce a waxy substance which traps dirt and protects the ear drum from infection. We are told not to poke cotton buds into our ears to clean out this wax but many people still do. Filling the ears with water can also be a problem as it can remain in the ear and affect the hearing for a while. Using a flannel around the entrance to the ear is probably the most useful way to keep it clean.

We enclose our feet in shoes and socks most of the time and the warmth and dampness encourages the growth of yeast or athlete's foot. The skin cracks between the toes and becomes red and itchy. The best way to avoid this is to wear cotton socks, wash your feet regularly, use an antifungal spray if you do have an infection and change shoes and socks regularly.

Humans are very prone to parasitic infestations, the main ones being head lice, pubic lice and intestinal worms. These are easily treated by modern chemicals.

9. PARASITIC, BACTERIAL, VIRAL, YEAST AND MOULD INFECTIONS

> *A third of a pillow could be made up of bugs, dead skin, dust mites and their faeces*

Our planet is teaming with life. Virtually everything in and upon it is covered in life in some form or other – even rocks in the hottest deserts and ice in the coldest climates have some kind of basic life in them. The air we breathe is full of bacteria, viruses, mould spores and plant seeds and we have evolved to cope with them. Most of them are harmless, because we have antibodies to kill them or our bodies are not suitable for their growth. Even when they do invade, our immune system makes antibodies, within a few days of infection, and kills them off.

Parasites have always been a problem, both for humans and the rest of the animal and plant kingdom. Many parasites merely feed off us, but don't kill us. It wouldn't be in their interests to do that because they would eventually run out of food. So-called civilized races have learnt how to deal with parasites, unlike the people of poorer countries whose lives are blighted by intestinal worms, blood sucking creatures and other nasty infestations.

Despite our vigilance, we are still prone to infestations, the most common being head lice and dust mites. Head lice can be killed with insecticide shampoo but dust mites are difficult to eradicate. Most of us are not unduly bothered by them, it is only those with severe asthma who need to have special bedding, high powered, filtered vacuum cleaners and a dust free living environment.

Always leave your bed covers turned down throughout the day to allow perspiration to evaporate – it is the damp environment that helps dust mites to thrive. Change your pillow regularly as well – after a couple of years your pillow could become sheltered housing for millions of mites and their detritus – ugh!

Although threadworms only live for about 5-6 weeks in the gut, before they die, the female worms lay tiny eggs around the anus. These cause itching around the back passage resulting in itching. When scratched the eggs get on the fingers and under the nails. These then get swallowed and the cycle continues.

Threadworm eggs can survive for up to two weeks outside the body. They get everywhere, in the bedding, flannels, towels etc. When someone in the house gets threadworm the rest of the family need to be treated as well.

Bacterial infections can become a serious problem if they manage to get a hold on your body. Fortunately our immune systems are pretty good, within a few days, at making the specific antibodies to fight each new invasion, but sometimes we need a helping hand. Antibiotics were thought to be the answer to every bacterial invasion, but the bacteria are mutating and becoming resistant and we are rapidly running out of effective antibiotics to treat serious, life threatening infections.

Bacteria are present everywhere and we have adapted to live alongside them. In fact they are frequently beneficial – we couldn't live without them in our gut where they help to break down our food and release vitamins. It is thought that we are in fact being too clean – by disinfecting everything, our children are no longer exposed to germs at an early age and so their immune systems are not adequately primed. Some auto-immune diseases, like arthritis and eczema are thought to be triggered by our immune systems, which start attacking our bodies instead of bacterial invaders.

One amazing discovery was made some years ago, concerning a bacteria called Helicobacter pylori, and its link to stomach ulcers and stomach cancer. Although more than 50% of the world's population harbour H. pylori in their upper gastrointestinal tract, some people are unlucky enough to be adversely affected by it. It burrows into the lining of the stomach and erodes the stomach wall away, causing pain and potentially life threatening bleeding.

In some cases this ulceration develops into stomach cancer. Scientist have developed the specific antibiotics to cure this, even if it has developed into cancer.

Viruses are tiny bundles of genetic material - either DNA or RNA - carried in a protein shell. They can't reproduce on their own – they need to invade a living cell. They are so small they can only be seen with an electron microscope. The DNA in a virus hijacks a cell, and uses it as a factory to make thousands of copies of itself.

Viral infections cannot be treated with antibiotics but our immune systems can still defend us from their invasion. Colds and flu are viral infections but because they mutate so readily into so many strains, we can't build up antibodies to them. Killer viruses, like polio, are now almost eliminated in the western world, with immunisation.

Yeasts are a large group of single celled fungi a few species of which are commonly used to make bread and alcoholic beverages. Most yeasts are harmless but one, Candida albicans, which normally lives harmlessly in the human gut, can become aggressive if we have a refined, high sugar diet. It feeds on the sugar, smothers friendly bacteria, punctures the gut lining and allows ethanol and partly digested food particles into the bloodstream.

Many women are aware of Thrush (candida albicans), an uncomfortable infection of the vagina. It causes soreness and itching and can make life miserable. Candida in the gut can cause all sorts of health problems, from allergies to join pain, brain fog to depression. If you have a high sugar, low fibre diet you need to think about Candida and its long-term side effects.

Moulds belong to the family of mushrooms and yeasts, and are collectively called fungi. They exist virtually everywhere and they break down organic material and recycle nutrients for plant life to use. They have an essential part to play – some plants can't survive without them but in our homes they can be deadly. If you have dampness in your home, moulds will thrive, living on organic material, such as wallpaper and destroying it. They release spores and waste products, which travel through the air, carrying with them mycotoxins and allergens.

Some people are sensitive to mould spores, which can cause nasal stuffiness, eye irritation, wheezing, or skin irritation. People who are already ill can suffer fever and shortness of breath. It can even grow in their lungs, causing respiratory diseases.

If you have mould in your home, try and increase the ventilation, reduce the dampness and treat any outbreaks with a bleach solution (1 cup bleach to a gallon of water.) There are plenty of de-humidifiers on the market, which do a good job of drying the building. I use one regularly in the winter, for a couple of hours a day, and regularly collect a pint of water each day. This water comes from breathing, kettles, cooking and clothes drying and is virtually impossible to stop, especially in the winter when all the windows are kept shut.

ABOUT THE AUTHOR

Sasha Craig-Taylor lives in Buckinghamshire, England and has been a remedial therapist for many years, working mainly with massage, manipulation, energy lamps and natural healing. Using these techniques she works with people suffering from stress related pain.

She has been advocating nutrition as a pathway to healing, for many years, and has written and published many articles on the subject, as well as being a public speaker.

Apart from her interest in remedial therapies and nutrition, Sasha is also an artist, writer and musician.

Also by this author:

Romantic Massage (a step by step guide for lovers of all ages)
ISBN-13: 978-1477551127

Why Sugar Makes You Hungry and Dieting Makes You Fat
ISBN-13: 978 1477450680

Billy's Daylight Boy (children's fiction)
ISBN-13: 978-1480164574

The Denniford Abduction (crime fiction)
ISBN-13: 978-1479348107

The Post-it Note (romance fiction)
ISBN-13: 978-1479236275

Kiss and Don't Tell (romance fiction)
ISBN-13: 978-1481081856

If you enjoy reading, visit:
www.a2zidx.com/more.php?books

www.ingramcontent.com/pod-product-compliance
Ingram Content Group UK Ltd.
Pitfield, Milton Keynes, MK11 3LW, UK
UKHW020139250726
13967UKWH00002B/752

9 781482 064087